Practical Child Psychiatry:
The clinician's guide

Bryan Lask

Professor of Child and Adolescent Psychiatry, St George's Hospital Medical School, University of London, London, UK and Huntercombe Hospital, Maidenhead, UK

Sharon Taylor

Specialist Registrar in Child Psychiatry, Academic Unit of Child and Adolescent Psychiatry, Imperial College of Science, Technology and Medicine, St Mary's Campus, London, UK

Kenneth P Nunn

Professor of Child Psychiatry, University of Newcastle and Director of Inpatient Child Psychiatry, John Hunter Hospital, Newcastle, New South Wales, Australia

© BMJ Publishing Group 2003
BMJ Books is an imprint of the BMJ Publishing Group

First published in 2003
by BMJ Books, BMA House, Tavistock Square,
London WC1H 9JR

www.bmjbooks.com

British Library Cataloguing in Publication Data

A catalogue record for this book is available from the British Library

ISBN 0 7279 1593 2

Typeset by SIVA Math Setters, Chennai, India
Printed and bound in Spain by Graphycems, Navarra

Contents

Preface

This book is written for the busy clinician who sees children and adolescents in distress. It aims to offer a practical guide to the assessment and treatment of emotional and behavioural problems, however they may present. Throughout we have tried to offer a perspective that will be of immediate value to the busy clinician. We have deliberately avoided learned theoretical discussions, slavish adherence to disease classification, and exhaustive reviews of the literature. Rather we have aimed to imagine ourselves in the clinics of the busy clinician and addressed what we believe to be of most relevance.

The first section offers a bird's eye view of psychiatric disorders, including definitions, demography, aetiology, and assessment. Section II describes the clinical picture of the more common disorders and overviews their treatment. The finer details of the most commonly used treatments are presented in section III.

We hope that this book will be of interest and value to all those working with troubled children and adolescents, whatever their professional background and regardless of their level of experience. However it is not for those who want a learned critique of the literature nor a detailed review of the very latest research findings. There are many other texts for such purposes. For an exhaustive and scholarly overview of the literature we suggest Rutter *et al.* or Noshpitz. For a developmental perspective use Graham *et al.* Practical advice on treatment planning can be found in Klykylo *et al.* For those sitting specialist exams Goodman and Scott and for those working in primary care Spender *et al.* will be of interest. But for busy clinicians who want a concise, practical, and accessible guide to the assessment and treatment of the child in distress we hope this book will be just what they need.

Further reading

Goodman R, Scott S. *Child psychiatry*. Oxford: Blackwell Science, 1997.
Graham P, Turk J, Verhulst F. Development and developmental psychopathology. In: *Child psychiatry: a developmental approach*. Oxford: Oxford Medical Publications/Oxford University Press, 1999.

Klykylo WM, Kay J, Rube D. *Clinical child psychiatry.* Philadelphia: WB Saunders, 1998.

Noshpitz J. *Handbook of child & adolescent psychiatry.* Chichester: John Wiley, 1997.

Rutter M, Taylor E, Hersov L. *Child and adolescent psychiatry. Modern approaches,* 3rd edn. Oxford: Blackwell Science, 1994.

Spender Q, Salt N, Dawkins J, Kenderick T, Hill P. *Child mental health in primary care.* Oxford: Radcliffe Medical Press, 2001.

Foreword

As knowledge in the specialties of medicine has expanded, textbooks have become longer in length and often narrower in focus so that authors can provide more in depth discussions of the various aspects of diseases included in the specialty. At the same time, clinicians practicing medicine seem to have less time to read for a variety of reasons, including the increase in administrative duties and paper work, seeing patients with more complicated problems, the need to help patients get appropriate services, and the frequent pressure to see ever more patients. What these busy clinicians often need is not another textbook focused on diseases, but rather a textbook focused on the practice of medicine.

Practical Child Psychiatry: The clinician's guide by three eminent child psychiatrists from two different continents is just that book for the busy mental health clinician. The authors provide the reader with a guide to caring for children and adolescents with mental health problems. The authors' focus is on the actual work of seeing patients and providing care, from the initial assessment to the treatment of the child and family. In this book, sections I and III, which cover the topics of assessment and treatment, offer much practical advice both to the trainee and the seasoned clinician. The authors provide many helpful suggestions about what to do, how to think and behave, and what pitfalls to avoid. Much of this information is encapsulated in the form of short lists and outlines, which provide an excellent starting point for examining one's style of practice and clinical work. Reading these lists will remind the reader of various patients and, perhaps, of some successes and failures. For me, these lists also are a reminder of the challenges of providing quality mental health care and how helpful such summaries can be in highlighting effective and ineffective care.

Section II provides 18 chapters on common clinical problems related to children's behaviours and emotions. For each problem, the authors provide a brief review, which addresses the salient clinical issues related to making the correct diagnosis. The chapters are focused on types of symptoms and conditions, rather than diseases; thus, the chapter on disruptive behaviours (chapter 5) helps the reader distinguish between ADHD (Attention Deficit Hyperactivity Disorder), CD (Conduct Disorder), and ODD (Oppositional Defiant Disorder). Chapters also are included on common problems of child health, such as child maltreatment, enuresis and encopresis, and medical illness.

A striking feature of this book is that much of the advice and recommendations are not, strictly speaking, supported by evidence-based medicine. While evidence-based medicine can provide data about the use of certain diagnostic tests or whether a certain medication or procedure is helpful for a specific condition, data from clinical trials are unlikely to inform how a clinician interacts with a patient, makes clinical decisions for the individual patient's problems, or provides the humanistic or therapeutic aspects of care.[1] What is extraordinarily helpful about this book is that the advice and recommendations are from experts who have extensive experience as clinicians and teachers. The reader, therefore, is getting advice that has been practiced, assessed, and revised. This is the best kind of information to help fill the large void left by all the questions that cannot or will not be answered through evidence-based medicine.

Lask, Nunn, and Taylor challenge the clinician to practice medicine in a more thoughtful, self-reflective manner. Their goal of improving the mental health care of children, adolescents, and families can be reached if the reader attends to the many pearls of wisdom in this book and translates these into effective practice.

A well known American child psychiatrist, Robert Coles wrote "A clinician must try to see what is strong as well as what is weak, what is sound as well as what ails, what might be struggling for expression in a person's life as well as what is lacking".[2] *Practical Child Psychiatry: The clinician's guide* will help clinicians provide better care by seeing the strengths and weaknesses of their patients and families.

1. Leventhal JM. Editorial: A continuing theme of taking stock – Clinical challenges for the new millennium. *Clinical Child Psychology and Psychiatry* 2000;5:309–311.
2. Coles R. *The South Goes North: Volume III of Children in Crisis.* Boston: Little, Brown and Co., 2000, p ix.

John M Leventhal, MD
Professor of Pediatrics and Child Study Center
Department of Pediatrics
Yale University School of Medicine
Connecticut, USA

Acknowledgements

The authors would like to thank Judith, Gideon and Adam Lask; Sev (Dr Mark Stickland, remembered with love); Rhonda, Daniel and Oliver Nunn; Ruth and Laurence Taylor; our colleagues; and most importantly our patients from whom we have learned so much.

Section I
A bird's eye view

1: Background

This chapter sets the context for the rest of the book by introducing the concept of psychiatric disorder, its demography and aetiology. The definition of psychiatric disorder is highly problematic (see below) and there are a large number of children whose symptoms or behaviour may not fulfil the criteria but nonetheless are troubled, distressed, or dysfunctional. We shall not discriminate against them in this book simply because they have failed to achieve a relatively arbitrary definition of a generally immeasurable and certainly intangible concept.

We do accept the need for diagnosis whenever possible, if only as a means of communication. But we will not be constrained by the monolithic classification schema (DSM and ICD) which seek to classify and categorise human distress. With these provisos we shall proceed.

What is psychiatric disorder?

Whenever the term "disorder" is used the concept of order is implied. With order, comes the notion of normality. For some, normality is a statistical concept in which the individual for any given factor falls within two standard deviations from the mean. Of course, there are those who fall outside two standard deviations in a beneficial way, for example a genius, a great athlete, or a brilliant leader. For others, normality has to do with the absence of disease. This begs the question of what is a disease? Some see this as simply the presence of structural abnormality at an anatomical level. Tattoos become diseases under this definition, whilst early hypertension may not.

It is difficult to use any definition of normality that does not invoke another concept, such as health, dysfunction, or deviation, which are equally problematic. In fact, the World Health Organisation has consistently had difficulty defining what is a disease. Psychiatric classifications have used the term disorder to avoid the problem of absence of disruption of anatomy and physiology in psychiatry.

Despite the difficulties in identifying the essential nature of a disorder, there are recurrent themes in each of the major classifications, which most clinicians recognise as central to the concept of disorder. These include: a subjective element—distress, and an objective or observed element—dysfunction. These two elements are qualified by the following characteristics: persistence, pervasiveness, and severity.

Thus psychiatric disorder is characterised by distress and dysfunction, which is persistent, pervasive, and severe. The particular nature of the distress and dysfunction together with the degree of persistence, pervasiveness and severity will identify the subcategory of the disorder.

A helpful way of thinking about whether distress and dysfunction constitute psychiatric disorder is to consider duration of time. Most people can be distressed or dysfunctional for several days without this being considered abnormal. For practical purposes, people can be impaired for three days or less without others becoming convinced that something should be done about it. If a problem persists for three weeks we would be alerted to the possibility that a disorder may be emerging. If difficulties persist for three months it is difficult to avoid the conclusion that something is wrong. A three year history of almost any problem is good evidence of long term dysfunction or chronicity.

A commonplace example of this is the response to grief. Most people might be completely stunned for three days following the death of a loved one. Although memories may remain for years, many people begin to recover from the profound emotional and physiological impact of bereavement after three weeks and are usually returning to normal function by three months. If grief persists at an intense level for three years it is likely that an abnormal grief process is in train and would probably be labelled "unresolved grief". There are other analogous life events, with very similar response patterns and a variety of individual differences.

Children are characterised by a marked dependency on the context within which they are cared for. Disorder, then, is not simply the categorisation of the individual, but a statement about how they are in relation to their environment. This has made the description of psychiatric disorder in childhood confusing. For instance, some clinicians use the term "child abuse" as if it were a diagnosis. Child abuse is an event or an ongoing statement of how a child is being treated. It does not indicate how the child responds, or what impact the abuse has on the child. From the child's point of view it is best to see child abuse as a predicament rather than a disorder. "Illness" or "disease" may best be used to describe those conditions where there are anatomical and physiological indices of disruption; "disorder" to delineate the response of the child to the disease; and "predicament" to describe the contextual constraints upon the child.

Conversely there are some children who are clearly disordered, but are not distressed. Children with brain damage, some children with attention deficit hyperactivity disorder (ADHD) and some forms of pervasive developmental disorder may not be distressed. Many of these children will cause distress in those who care for them. There are some children who are extremely distressed but continue to function in all domains to the satisfaction of those around. However, the level of their distress has a negative impact in its own right because of the distress it evokes within others. Clearly there is no completely satisfactory definition of psychiatric disorder, particularly in childhood, nor for that matter of disease. We might conclude however that whilst it is difficult to define an elephant, it is easy to recognise one!

For practical purposes we have therefore chosen to define psychiatric disorder as "A condition characterised by distress and dysfunction in the child, which is persistent in time, pervasive across each domain of experience and severe in degree, but is not limited to social deviance or disadvantage alone."

What sort of disorders do children experience?

Each part of a child's experience has the potential for distress and dysfunction. A child's feelings form the basis for emotional disorders. A child's behaviour forms the basis for disruptive disorders. A child's development may be impaired globally, as in the pervasive developmental disorders, or focally, as in the specific learning disorders. A child's thinking may be disordered in psychosis and a child's bodily experience may be distorted leading to somatisation disorder. In general in childhood there is a tendency towards comorbidity, i.e.

Table 1.1 Development of psychological problems

Age	Problems encountered
Neonates and babies	Feeding, sleep and crying
Toddlers 1–3 years	Motor activity, speech, bladder, bowel control, and temper tantrums
Preschoolers 3–5 years	As above, with fears and phobias, habit disorders, feeding and sleeping difficulties
Infant schoolers 5–7 years	All of the above plus separation anxiety and pervasive developmental disorders
Primary schools 7–8 years	Specific learning disorders and ADHD
Late primary school	Depression and anxiety
Early adolescence	Peer difficulties, conflict with parents, depression, sexuality and suicidality, eating disorders (restrictive), and social phobia
Mid to late adolescence	Depression, bipolar disorder and schizophrenia, bulimia, and substance abuse

mixtures of symptom patterns that are rarely mutually exclusive.

Within the emotional disorders, anxiety (especially separation anxiety) and depression are the most common. Within the disruptive disorders, oppositional defiant disorder, ADHD and conduct disorder are most frequent. Mixtures of the emotional disorders and disruptive disorders also commonly occur.

Other conditions include conversion disorders, somatisation disorders, eating disorders, obsessive compulsive disorder, tics, social phobia, the autistic spectrum disorders, and the major psychoses. Far more rarely dementia, delirium, and genetic disorders, which give rise to a behavioural phenotype, may occur. Table 1.1 summarises the more common disorders by age and a full presentation of the wide range of psychiatric disorder of childhood and adolescence is provided in Section II.

Demographic considerations

How many children suffer with psychiatric disorder? We do not know. Most research studies find that between 10% and 20% of children at any one time have distress and dysfunction which clinicians would rate as a disorder. However it is likely that there are many more children who have emotional or behavioural problems which do not fulfil criteria for a diagnosis of psychiatric disorder. Such situations are sometimes described as "subclinical".

Lifetime prevalence of psychiatric disorder will naturally be higher than point prevalence, with a significant number of young people moving from "normal" or "subclinical" status to overt psychiatric disorder and back again over time.

What about gender distribution? Prior to puberty the balance of psychiatric disorder is more heavily weighted towards boys due to their high incidence of disruptive disorder. After puberty the balance steadily sways towards girls bearing the greater burden of disorder due to a steady rise in depression and anxiety. The overall assessment of the rate of psychiatric disorder rarely takes into account risk taking behaviour, accident proneness, and juvenile criminality. When these factors, together with the increase in substance abuse in males, are taken into account, it is unlikely that females would predominate in the burden of morbidity.

Causation

Causation is best conceptualised using two complementary models: (a) the biopsychosocial model and (b) the "3Ps", i.e. predisposing, precipitating, and perpetuating factors.

The biopsychosocial model

In this model due consideration is given to the roles of biological, psychological and social factors. Each is likely to contribute but the relative significance will vary from one disorder to another. For example in attention deficit disorder, biological factors such as neurotransmitter imbalance are likely to have a major influence, but psychological factors such as the child's temperament, and social factors such as styles of parenting, are also likely to contribute. In school refusal psychological factors such as poor self esteem, and social factors such as peer group teasing or bullying, may be predominant, but biological factors such as a genetic predisposition toward anxiety may be a necessary prerequisite.

The 3 Ps

This model acknowledges the relative contribution of: predisposing factors, precipitating factors, and perpetuating factors.

Predisposing factors

These are the factors that are a necessary prerequisite for the development of a specific disorder. In the absence of such factors that particular disorder cannot occur. There are two main types of predisposing factors: biological and environmental.

Biological An increasing number of psychiatric disorders have been shown to have a genetic or biological contribution. However, unlike the early studies of single gene mutations it is increasingly obvious that many of the disorders in psychiatry represent functional polymorphisms of traits that might be adaptive in different environments. Large numbers of loci representing genes of small effect might combine to interact with the environment in order to give rise to the final phenotype. Genetics no longer should be portrayed as deterministic. It may well be that in the future, genetic factors will be more modifiable than environmental contributions.

- *Chronic medical illness.* Repeated studies have shown an increase in psychiatric morbidity associated with chronic medical illness in childhood. Children with systemic disease not involving the central nervous system usually have two to three times the rate of psychiatric disorder. Children with chronic disease of the central nervous system will have five to six times the rate of psychiatric disorder. Multifocal lesions of the central nervous system will have greater morbidity than unifocal lesions. Seizure active lesions will have greater morbidity. Those children with complex partial seizures are more likely to have increased rates of psychiatric morbidity compared to those with generalised tonic clonic seizures and absence seizures. Secondary depression is common with diseases such as diabetes, ulcerative colitis, and severe asthma.

- *Specific developmental disorder.* Children with both expressive and receptive language disorders are more likely to have psychiatric difficulties. Those with receptive disorders are more likely to have associated social impairment than those with expressive disorders. Children with specific reading, mathematics or other learning disorders have an increased rate of emotional and behavioural disturbance.
- *Intellectual impairment.* Children with mild intellectual impairment often have comorbid psychiatric disorder. Because their intellectual disability is mild, it is apt to be overlooked. Those with moderate to severe disability have the greatest burden of comorbid psychiatric disorder, while those who are profoundly intellectually disabled are generally too impaired physically to be behaviourally disturbed.

Environmental   The society or environment in which we live may predispose to various psychiatric disorders; for example, anorexia nervosa (see chapter 8) tends only to occur in societies where thinness is valued and obesity disparaged—predominantly societies in which food is plentiful. By contrast, children brought up in a deprived and chaotic environment may be predisposed to disruptive disorders (see chapter 15).

Precipitating factors

These are the factors that trigger the onset of the disorder and include parenting styles, other environmental factors, and specific cognitions.

Parenting styles
- *Overprotection.* This is particularly common in the emotional disorders such as depression and anxiety, but also in more extreme form may be found in those children

with somatisation disorder. Overprotection in the extreme may be as damaging as abuse or neglect. An example of this would be a situation in which a parent is so overprotective that the child is socially isolated. In chronic life threatening conditions overprotection may prolong or complicate an illness.

- *Dissatisfaction and criticism.* Parental dissatisfaction and criticism have been shown to be key factors in the emergence of both emotional and disruptive disorders. Clearly they can vary in intensity. For example, compare: (a) a parent shouting at a child on one occasion "I'm fed up with you doing that!'; (b) repeated comments of that nature; (c) "I'm fed up with you doing that, you're an idiot!"; (d) "I'm fed up with you doing that, you're an idiot! You always have been an idiot and you always will be an idiot!"; and (e) "I'm fed up with you doing that, you're an idiot! You always have been an idiot and you always will be an idiot! Get out of here!" The more intense and frequent the criticism the more that child is at risk.
- *Parental personality difficulties or psychiatric disorder.* It may at first seem obvious that children, who are exposed to the symptoms of their disturbed parents, may themselves become ill. However, the situation is not always straightforward. Some parents, particularly depressed mothers, often take steps to protect children from their symptoms. Other parents are so obviously ill that their children can identify when they are sick and when they are well, and respond to them appropriately. Surprisingly, those parents who are most likely to have a negative impact on their children are neither the psychotic nor the profoundly depressed, but those with longstanding personality difficulties and problems in interpersonal relationships. Children may find it difficult to identify their parents as ill when their parents have life long personality problems. Another explanation relates to the coping style of many parents with personality difficulties which may cause children to believe that they are the cause of their parent's problems. For example, when a parent denies any responsibility when things go wrong and blames the children for causing the problem, children are likely to believe their parents. Further, if the parents see the

world in rigid, black and white terms, in which those who agree with them are good and those who disagree are bad, the children are likely to employ problem solving techniques which involve "either/or" thinking instead of the capacities of compromise and negotiation.

- *Marital discord.* Marital discord has consistently been shown to be associated with increased rates of psychiatric disorder in children. Those marriages where the discord is open, overtly conflictual and enlists the children in the conflict, are more likely to lead to psychiatric disorder than those marriages where the discord is covert and the failure in the relationship is essentially apathetic. That is to say, a marriage where there is a lack of relationship between the partners is less distressing to the children than those marriages which are actively conflictual. Assessing the quality of a marriage involves taking into account both the presence of negative factors, such as discord and dissatisfaction, and the absence of positive factors such as warmth expressed between partners and satisfaction with one another. Children frequently attribute to themselves responsibility for parental fighting and the breakdown of marital relationships.

Other environmental factors These include peer group difficulties, school-based problems, and adverse life events. Such factors in isolation cannot precipitate a disorder, but within the context of specific predisposing factors they may act as triggers. For example teenage girls with anorexia nervosa may have been teased about being overweight. However the vast majority of teenage girls who are teased in this way do not subsequently develop anorexia nervosa. The teasing can only trigger the disorder within the context of the predisposing factors.

Specific cognitions Over the last 20 years, specific thinking patterns have been increasingly proposed as causative elements in the emergence of mood disorder and problems of impulsivity. For example the tendency to believe that adversity will be **permanent** and **pervasive** and to **personalise** the origins of the adversity may precipitate depression. Permanency can be seen as a "Humpty Dumpty" phenomenon in which when things go wrong, they are seen as irreversible. Pervasiveness might be illustrated by the "House of Cards" phenomenon in which when one card falls they all do. One thing goes wrong and the child feels that everything is wrong. Personalisation is illustrated by the tendency in all situations to say either explicitly or implicitly "It's all my fault" or "this doesn't happen to other people".

Perpetuating factors

These are the factors that maintain a disorder once it has emerged; for example, a child with tics may be teased at school and the ensuing distress leads to further tics and a vicious cycle is thus set in place.

As with precipitating factors the perpetuating factors may be biological, psychological, or social; for example, the child may have a predisposition to develop tics and the onset of these is precipitated by bullying at school. They may be perpetuated by the biological predisposition, teasing at school (social), and poor self esteem and social skills (psychological).

Summary of causation

The biopsychosocial and the "3Ps" models are generally sufficient to formulate a working understanding of the development and maintenance of most child psychiatric disorders. Predisposing, precipitating and perpetuating factors are all likely to contribute and each of these may be biological, social or psychological. Often there is considerable overlap. Consider the teenage girl with anorexia nervosa. The predisposing factors are likely to include a genetic (biological) component/sensitivity and a particular personality type (psychological), as well as the powerful influence of society's preoccupation with the ideal of thinness. Precipitating factors might include the onset of puberty (biological), teasing about being overweight (social), and poor self esteem (psychological). The illness may be perpetuated by the effects of starvation impairing insight (biological), the sense of achievement through weight loss (psychological), and inconsistent parental management and peer group envy (social).

Conclusion

Child psychiatry requires a "first principles" approach to a much greater degree than almost any other field of clinical work. Diagnostic categories rarely provide a key to understanding mechanisms of disease or causation. The conditions are common, the factors contributing blend imperceptibly into "way of life" and "human condition" issues. It is understandable therefore that many people have a view, and some very strong views, on the causes and cures for children's troubles. Some of these involve changing society. This book does not address these issues. Some involve reiterating what parents ought to do. It is remarkable how unproductive such a seemingly straightforward approach is in clinical practice, although preventive education for parents does offer exciting possibilities. In this book we focus on helping a child and family who are already experiencing difficulties and on the practical solutions.

Section II of this book provides a detailed description of the common (and some not so common) psychiatric problems of childhood and adolescence and Section III describes their management.

Further reading

Cantwell D, Rutter M. Classification—conceptual issues and substantive findings. In: Rutter M, Taylor E, Hersov L, eds. *Child and adolescent psychiatry—a developmental approach*. Oxford: Blackwell, 1995:3–21.

Nunn K, Nicholls D, Lask B. A new taxonomy—the Uluru personal experiential profile. *Clinical Child Psychology and Psychiatry* 2000;5:313–27.

2: Assessment

The key to a full understanding of the child's problems is establishing a good rapport and undertaking a comprehensive assessment. This chapter focuses on these essentials. Success in this first meeting will largely be determined by gaining the confidence of the child and parents. Each clinician has his or her own strategies for creating rapport and there is no one correct way. We choose to ensure a child-friendly environment, privacy, tranquility, and as much time as possible. We always introduce ourselves and greet each person individually. It is far preferable to avoid "white coats" (they are still worn by some doctors, though fortunately few, who work with children) and equally preferable to avoid sitting behind a large desk, not unknown in some medical settings. Irrespective of the underlying problems, most children and families will require some time given to listening to and exploring the symptoms.

Establishing rapport

One of the most important and potentially difficult tasks for any of us who work with children and adolescents is that of talking with them. However most clinicians will be familiar with the scenario of failing to communicate with a shy, frightened, angry or withdrawn youngster. So how do we talk with children and adolescents, and especially when they don't particularly want to talk with us? A number of important considerations apply:

- *The context.* Privacy is always desirable and sometimes essential. Children cannot be expected to talk about personal, worrying or upsetting matters, nor to listen to and understand complex explanations, if there are frequent interruptions or other distractions, or if they can be overheard. A quiet room with well equipped and age appropriate play and drawing materials facilitate the process.

- *Who should be present?* This depends on the age and wishes of the child, and the purposes of the meeting. Younger children will want and may need a parent or other trusted adult, while older children are more likely to vary in their wishes, and teenagers should certainly be given the opportunity to talk on their own.
- *Talking is a two way process.* Any communication is interactional. If talking is to be useful, it must include listening. Listening involves not only hearing what is said, but also how is it said, i.e. volume and tone of voice, body posture, eye contact, and facial expression.
- *Approach and attitude.* This should be relaxed and friendly. The discussion should always start with a neutral and non-threatening topic, and the clinician should be guided throughout by the child's responses. Imagination and creativity will help overcome many reservations.
- *The means of communication.* Talking with children involves far more than words. Play, toys and drawings provide a very fruitful means of communication.
- *Strategies.* When reticence prevails, children can be helped to overcome this by the means of various techniques. These include:
  - 'Generalising', i.e. making a facilitative statement that gives the message that many people of the child's age have this problem
  - Identification, i.e. use of one's own experiences
  - Musing, i.e. thinking aloud about what might be troubling the child
  - Pre-empting, i.e. when a child or adolescent is likely to be determinedly silent, express the expectation that he or she will be silent and that is okay.
- *Idioms, stories, metaphors and magic.* Upsetting thoughts and feelings can be explored indirectly. Stories, dreams, metaphors, and wishes offer simple and enjoyable techniques for engaging children in difficult topics.

The outcome is likely to be rewarding if the setting is right, and the sensitive and imaginative clinician adapts language and medium of communication to the current developmental level, avoids leading questions or statements, and listens carefully.

A comprehensive assessment

In keeping with the model of aetiology outlined in chapter 1, a comprehensive assessment involves paying due attention to biological, psychological and social factors, and to predisposing, precipitating and perpetuating factors.

Assessment of the child and family

There is no best way of conducting an assessment. A wide range of factors will determine whether to start by seeing the whole family together, both parents and child, one parent and child, the parents alone, or the child alone. When assessing young children it is more appropriate to have at least one parent present for the first meeting, whereas adolescents generally prefer to be seen alone. Ideally when both parents are available they should be seen together. It is wise to give all parties as much choice as possible in deciding on such matters. We offer below a suggested outline of an interview with the child, parents, and other members of the family. However flexibility and practicality are paramount in order to be helpful. A more detailed discussion of interviewing and treating families is covered in chapter 22. Specific issues relating to each group of disorders are raised in the relevant chapters.

Following greetings and introductions, the initial assessment should include obtaining demographic details such as names, ages, schools, and occupations.

A useful question thereafter is: "What are some of the concerns you have had that made you decide to come here today?" This allows for exploration of the concerns including their development, duration, and frequency, precipitating, perpetuating and relieving factors, what has and has not helped, effect on the rest of the family, and desired outcome. At some point it is important to explore the child's developmental, educational and medical history and the family history.

Particular questions can be helpful in exploring a specific diagnosis; for example, "Has Robert ever had any unusual movements in his body, on his face, or limbs?" might be a very specific probe for tics.

"Is there a difference in William's behaviour between when he is with other children or just alone with you?" might explore problems specific to a particular situation in a child with attention difficulties.

"Have you ever thought Jacky was acting as if someone was speaking to her when there was no one with her?" might elicit the internal preoccupation and external behaviour associated with hallucinations. Again this might be followed up either in the family or individually with, "Have you sometimes heard people speaking to you but you couldn't be sure whether there was anyone there?"

"Has there been an actual loss of Alison's abilities or just a drop-off when compared to others her own age?" is a quite complex question trying to explore the possibility of developmental delay versus dementia. This might be followed up by a direct question to Alison, "Are there things that you can't do now Alison that you could do before?"

Questions exploring suicidality, dangerousness, abuse, and sexuality are often more productive in the individual interview.

Pulling together the different threads

Before the end of the meeting it is important to attempt a tentative statement about the possibilities as to the nature of the problem and what needs to be done. Ample time should be provided for questions and discussion. A simple statement of when there will be another meeting and what will be its purpose may help allay anxieties. Opportunity to make contact in the meantime should be encouraged because parents often think of things they wished to say or ask after leaving.

It is worth checking whether what is being offered matches the expectations of the family and whether any new concerns have arisen as a result of the meeting.

There is no clear dividing line between assessment and treatment, and ascertaining the effects of offering advice, reassurance, support and symptomatic relief add to the assessment process. In any event symptomatic relief of physical, psychological or interpersonal difficulties may be paramount in the first instance. Overwhelming anxiety may require medication. Headaches may require relaxation therapy. Interpersonal difficulties may require time apart and extra support from people outside the family. It is always a matter of judgment as to whether the provision of relief will undermine pursuing longer term definitive treatment. Experienced clinicians generally provide more support to start with and steadily address longer term issues as treatment progresses.

A broad overview of treatment is provided in chapter 21, the finer details of specific therapies in chapters 22–25, and the specific treatments for each disorder in the relevant chapters.

Further reading

Angold A. Clinical interviewing with children and adolescents. In: Rutter M, Taylor E, Hersov L, eds. *Child and adolescent psychiatry—a developmental approach.* Oxford: Blackwell, 1995:51–63.

Lask B. Talking with children. *British Journal of Hospital Medicine* 1992;**47**:688–71.

Section II
The clinical picture

3: Fears and anxieties

Introduction

Fear is feeling a sense of threat *in the presence of* a particular person, situation, or object. Anxiety is a feeling of threat experienced *in anticipation of* an undesirable event even if the specific nature of what may happen is not known. In practice, fears and anxieties are frequently intermingled. Anxiety can be considered either normal or abnormal depending on the context and degree of the anxiety. It becomes pathological when the fear is out of proportion to the context of the life situation and, in childhood, when it is out of keeping with the expected behaviour for the developmental stage of the child.

Developmental considerations

The normal development of anxiety

Younger children are able to relay only limited information about fears and anxieties. In the case of infants and toddlers, who are unable to talk about emotions, it is assumed that they may experience fears. Their limited capacity to conceptualise the future may protect them from at least some anxieties. However, infants can be observed to respond to the emotions of the persons holding them.

The development of object constancy, that is the ability to hold parents in mind even when they are absent, occurs at around 7–8 months. At this time fear emerges with strangers, when in new situations, or when separated from a familiar person such as the child's mother. This fear of strangers and separation anxiety peaks at about 18 months and then becomes less intense with occasional peaks with the commencement of preschool and school, illness, or family adversity.

In early childhood, between 3 and 5 years old, fears also appear in response to animals, darkness, the toilet, and imagined creatures and situations. Children may compensate or cope with these fears by seeing themselves as big, smart, brave, and strong. From 6 to 11 years fears of illness, parental death, personal embarrassment, failing at a task, and losing control are common. The death of a grandparent at this time will accentuate these concerns. Fear of being teased at school and disapproved of by the teacher may be prominent. This is a time of life when most children have to learn how to manage disappointments. Learning how to manage their anxiety about being chosen for the choir or sports team, being invited to someone's birthday party or to play and doing well in the annual Christmas play, all provide opportunities to negotiate the anxiety–disappointment cycle with parental support.

Adolescence heralds other interpersonal issues with a deep awareness of others of the same age group. Continual comparisons of bodies, clothing, material circumstances, behaviour, relationships, and family life, form the fabric of their thoughts, life, and conversations with each other. Emergence of fears of specific social settings and the fear of failing to appear and behave like everyone else is common.

The extent to which any of these fears will dominate individual children at each stage of development will depend on their temperament, life experiences, the parents' response to them, the child's level of understanding, and what the future holds for that particular child. Individual variations and exceptions to almost any behavioral formula are common.

Age related changes in circumstances that can provoke anxiety are paralleled by the onset of pathological anxieties. For example, separation anxiety begins in the preschool years, animal phobias begin in early childhood, performance anxiety in late childhood, and social anxiety in adolescence. Separation anxiety disorder may occur at any time after the attachment period, but typically occurs in late childhood and early adolescence. Anxieties are experienced in ways similar to adults with both mental and physical components (Figure 3.1). However, they are often more diffuse in their effects than in adults, more bound up in a non-articulated distress and therefore more often expressed with physical symptoms.

The following anxiety disorders will be considered in this chapter:

- Generalised anxiety disorder
- Specific phobias
- Social phobias

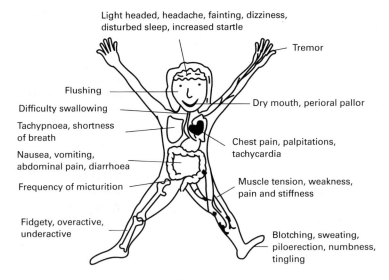

Light headed, headache, fainting, dizziness, disturbed sleep, increased startle

Tremor

Flushing

Difficulty swallowing

Tachypnoea, shortness of breath

Nausea, vomiting, abdominal pain, diarrhoea

Frequency of micturition

Fidgety, overactive, underactive

Dry mouth, perioral pallor

Chest pain, palpitations, tachycardia

Muscle tension, weakness, pain and stiffness

Blotching, sweating, piloerection, numbness, tingling

Figure 3.1 Physical symptoms of anxiety

- Separation anxiety disorders
- School refusal
- Panic disorder

Post-traumatic stress disorder and obsessive compulsive disorder are also usually categorised as anxiety disorders but are considered in other chapters (see chapters 4 and 9).

Epidemiology

Childhood anxiety disorders are one of the most common problems found in childhood. Estimates of prevalence vary from 0·9% to 8% (Table 3.1) Despite the high prevalence rates, the impairment produced and the good response to therapy, anxiety disorders are generally underrecognised and undertreated. Through childhood there is no gender predominance, but in late adolescence onwards females are affected more commonly. Rates increase in children living in social adversity and in inner city residents.

Table 3.1 The prevalence rates of specific anxiety disorders

Anxiety disorder	Prevalence rate	Reference
Generalised anxiety disorder	Six month prevalence rate 2–6%. No gender preference	Costello *et al.*[1] 1996 Verhulst *et al.*[2] 1997 Muris *et al.*[3] 1998
Specific phobias	2–3% though only a small percentage will seek treatment. More frequent in girls	Silverman *et al.*[4] 1993
Social phobias	0·9–1·1%. Girls more than boys	Klykylo *et al.*[5] 1998
Separation anxiety disorder (SAD)	4%. Up to 8% of children presenting to psychiatric clinic have SAD though will generally present as school refusal. More frequent in girls. Mean age at presentation 10 years	Last *et al.*[6] 1992
School refusal	1–2%. Peak age at times of school change, that is 5, 11 and 14–15 years	Weiner,[7] 1982
Panic disorder	5% in the 13–18 year community age group. Rare before puberty. Peak age of onset 15–19 years	Macaulary and Kleinknecht,[8] 1989

Aetiology

The development of anxiety disorders has a multifactorial basis.

Genetics

There are increased rates of anxiety disorder in the children of adults with anxiety disorders and in parents of children with anxiety disorders. Twin studies have shown that both genetics and non-shared environmental factors make equal contributions to the familiality of anxiety disorders.

Biology

Children who have inherited temperaments of behavioral inhibition, characterised by initial timidity, shyness, emotional restraint with unfamiliar people or contexts, are more prone to anxiety disorders. Neuroimaging has shown a reduced hippocampal volume in adult patients with chronic anxiety. Biological correlates in childhood panic disorders include blunted growth hormone response to noradrenergic challenges, which is also seen in childhood depression. In addition, adolescent girls with anxiety disorder have been noted to have abnormal growth patterns.

Learning theory

Maladaptive anxiety may occur as a learned behaviour following exposure to a frightening situation. The child learns that avoiding situations that evoke distress results in anxiety reduction, thus serving to reward the avoidance behaviour and so perpetuating it. Avoidance behaviour emerges as a consequence to escape from the dangerous situation. Anxiety could therefore be viewed as a distress avoidance syndrome.

Generalised anxiety disorder

This disorder is characterised by an unrealistic or excessive, persistent, generalised anxiety about everyday situations, occurring most days. It may be accompanied by restlessness, fatigue, poor concentration, muscle tension, other physical symptoms, and sleep disturbance. The anxiety or physical symptoms cause impairment in many areas of functioning, including socially and at school.

Clinical features

The preschool child

What distinguishes children with anxiety disorder from normal developmental anxiety is the intensity of the anxiety.

This is manifested by severe separation anxiety, irritability and tension, prolonged temper tantrums, and difficulties when going to sleep. The child may fail to settle at playschool or childcare after the departure of their parents and mix poorly with other children. New situations provoke distress and result in clingy behaviour with caregivers. At the same time specific fears may combine with separation anxiety to assume a dominating intensity. It becomes clear that it is not merely separation but the whole of the child's experience that is fraught with anxiety.

Children between 5 and 12 years

In this age group the anxiety is increasingly persistent and widespread with an average of six specific worries compared to one or two in normal children. The anxiety is difficult to control, interferes with daily activities, and is frequently mentioned. The content of these worries includes excessive concern about getting on with others and knowing what to do. There is an increased self-consciousness often with a need for constant reassurance. This may take the form of fear of embarrassment or ridicule. The child may have difficulty relaxing and somatic complaints with no organic origin are common, such as limb pains, headaches, abdominal pain, and recurrent cough (see also chapter 13).

Adolescents

In addition to the features seen in younger children, the anxiety may be accompanied by concerns about identity, the "meaning of life", personal appearance, physical health, and negative evaluation by others. Characteristically, there is excessive anxiety about everyday occurrences—"a general inability to cope". Everything seems to be problematic and parents find themselves trying but failing to shield their child from potential disappointments.

Treatment of generalised anxiety disorder

Treatment involves a combined approach of parental counselling (see chapter 22), cognitive behaviour therapy

(CBT; see chapter 24), and pharmacotherapy such as SSRIs (selective serotonin reuptake inhibitors), benzodiazepines, and buspirone (see chapter 25).

The busy clinician is wise to focus on slowly and surely moving towards a normal developmental trajectory rather than trying to find a deep significance to the anxiety. In the presence of intense parental anxiety, it is reasonable to note that this is a problem that affects more than one member of the family, and may have a genetic component. It is often helpful to be slow to criticise, quick to minimise guilt, and astute at emphasizing success.

Prognosis

The course is variable with a pattern of relapses and remissions with some continuation into adulthood.

Specific phobias

Specific fears are common in childhood with different fears emerging at different ages. The fear is described as a phobia when the feared event or object is avoided, daily function is impaired and the fear and avoidance persists.

The anxiety may be expressed by crying, tantrums, panic, freezing, or clinging. The child may or may not recognise the irrational nature of their fear, depending on cognitive capacity.

Clinical features

In most cases, the amount of impairment is mild, particularly if the feared situation is rarely encountered. Occasionally, the phobia can lead to the child's activities being curtailed and restricted. The nature of the phobias, as with normal fears, correlates with age. Examples of specific phobias include reactions to animals, darkness, and imaginary creatures in childhood; in adolescence fear of illness, death or war are more characteristic.

27

Treatment

The most useful approach is a combination of parental counselling (see chapter 22) and CBT (see chapter 24). It is important to inform the child and parent that avoidance increases the anxiety and exposure to the feared object reduces it.

Prognosis

In general, mild fears subside and severe phobias may persist into adulthood.

Social phobia: (social anxiety disorder)

Social phobia is an exaggeration and persistence of the normal phase of stranger anxiety, which occurs in children of up to 30 months of age. It is more than just shyness as it results in dysfunction and disrupted relationships. It is characterised by a marked and persistent fear of humiliation or embarrassment. Such situations are subsequently avoided or endured with intense anxiety. Exposure to feared social situations provokes anxiety, which may take the form of panic, crying, tantrums, freezing, withdrawl, and autonomic arousal such as sweating, palpitations, blushing, and tremor. Some such children are mute in specific situations although not in others, a condition known as "selective mutism". The child may or may not realise that the fear is excessive. The avoidance, anxious anticipation or distress interferes with the child's functioning, for example at school, social activities, or in relationships. The phobia may be to a specific situation or generalised across a number of different social or performance situations. Onset can occur either insidiously or following a particularly stressful or embarrassing event and may occur in any age group.

Treatment consists of a combination of parental counselling (see chapter 22), social skills training, and CBT (see chapter 24) with the occasional use of medication (see chapter 25). Both the child and family should be steadily and firmly encouraged not to avoid the feared situation. The smallest incursion into the social arena not previously attempted should be encouraged and rewarded. New gains should be consolidated before proceeding to the next step.

Prognosis

If left untreated the condition continues through into adult life. There is an increased risk of depression, substance abuse, and suicide. The frequency, gravity and persistence of comorbidity (see below) and complications make social phobia an important disorder to recognise and treat.

Separation anxiety

Separation anxiety is developmentally inappropriate, persisting and excessive anxiety concerning separation from home or from those to whom the child is attached, and causes significant distress or impairment in social, academic or other areas of functioning.

The onset may be either acute or insidious. It will often follow a stressful event such as illness or loss.

Young children (5–8 years old) are more likely to worry about something scary like a ghost or monster, or harm befalling their parents. Subsequently they find it hard to separate from a parent. They have problems attending school or sleeping away from home. Such children often have problems sleeping alone and will seek to be in the parental or a sibling's bed. Nightmares with themes of separation may be prominent.

At 9–12 years of age the child may experience severe distress on separation, becoming withdrawn, apathetic, sad, irritable, and socially withdrawn. Schoolwork and school attendance may be impaired and somatic complaints often occur.

The adolescent is most likely to experience physical symptoms, of which recurrent abdominal pain and headaches are the most common. Again school attendance and schoolwork are impaired. School refusal (see below) is often associated with separation anxiety.

Treatment involves a combination of parental counselling and family therapy (see chapter 22), liaison with the school, CBT (see chapter 24), and possibly SSRIs (see chapter 25).

Prognosis

This is generally good although it may persist into adult life, presenting as agoraphobia, anxiety, or depression.

School refusal

School refusal is best conceptualised as a symptom rather than a disorder. There can be many reasons for refusal to attend school, including separation anxiety (see above), family dysfunction, bullying, poor peer relationships, and academic underachievement. The term school phobia is often used synonymously with school refusal but should be reserved for those situations where the feared element is specifically within the school. Both terms need to be distinguished from truancy (see chapter 5) in which there is no anxiety about school attendance, but rather the child chooses to stay away from school, usually under peer group influence.

Clinical features

School refusal may present acutely or insidiously. Clinical features include behavioural symptoms such as determined refusal to leave home for school or increasing anxiety as school is approached, and physical symptoms such as poor appetite, headaches, nausea, vomiting, abdominal pains, and diarrhoea. The symptoms are particularly prominent in the morning and following a weekend or end of holiday. When physical symptoms are particularly prominent it is sometimes referred to as "masquerade syndrome".

Regardless of the causes, the reduction in anxiety by not being at school maintains the problem.

Treatment

The aim of treatment is to ascertain and resolve the underlying problems and help the child return to school. Treatment involves a combination of parental counselling (see chapter 22), liaison with the school, CBT, and anxiolytics (see chapter 25). A careful balance needs to be found between under- and overinvestigating physical symptoms. Early return to school is aimed for, often using a gradual approach. This would start with short visits to the school, but not necessarily going into the classroom. The visits can slowly be increased in length and intensity. It can be helpful if the child is accompanied by a friend. Clearly close collaboration with the school is necessary, and given how common school refusal is many schools have experience of how to manage it. The key is to redress the balance so that it is more rewarding to go to school than to stay at home. It is not advisable that the child receives home tuition for this increases the "comfort factor" at home and reduces the urgency for school return. Nor is the need for socialisation addressed by home schooling.

Prognosis

In general, mild and acute cases resolve with the appropriate treatment. The later the onset the harder it is to resolve the problem, and a small proportion develop anxiety or mood disorders in adult life.

Panic disorder

Panic disorder consists of recurrent unexpected panic attacks. These tend to be discrete episodes which begin abruptly, and consist of any of the following symptoms: palpitations, sweating, shaking, shortness of breath, choking, chest pain, abdominal distress, dizziness, feeling lightheaded or faint, derealisation or depersonalisation, paraesthesia, and fear of losing control or dying. The symptoms tend to reach a peak in 10 minutes. There may be no obvious precipitating factor.

Treatment

Treatment should involve a combination of parental counselling (see chapter 22), SSRIs (see chapter 25), and CBT (see chapter 24).

"Practising" panic attacks and using slow breathing to arrest the attack, moves the child and parent from passive and fearful anticipation to active mastery and confidence. Focus on relaxation, slow breathing and challenging catastrophic thought patterns during the attack may be useful. Slow breathing exercises are best practised when the child is calm.

Prognosis

The disorder has a good short term prognosis but may re-emerge intermittently and often at important developmental or personal times.

Comorbidity and differential diagnosis

Comorbidity takes two forms:

1. Different types of anxiety disorder may coexist, for example school refusal and panic attacks, or selective mutism and separation anxiety.
2. Other psychiatric disorders, including depression (see chapter 6), obsessive compulsive disorder (see chapter 3), post-traumatic stress disorder (see chapter 4), and disruptive disorders (see chapter 5).

The differential diagnosis includes all the comorbid disorders mentioned above.

Conclusion

The disorders of anxiety in childhood are common, distressing, and treatable, but often missed or left untreated. They are almost all associated with episodes of high arousal and avoidance behaviour. They are also frequently associated with medical symptoms, presage other psychiatric disorders, and are in danger of becoming chronic if allowed to go unchecked. Most improve with parental counselling, simple behavioural and cognitive approaches, and medication.

References

1 Costello EJ, Angold A, Burns BJ, *et al.* The Great Smoky Mountains Study of youth: goals, design, methods, and the prevalence of DSM-III-R disorders. *Archives of General Psychiatry* 1996;**53**:1129–36.
2 Verhulst FC, Van der Ende J, Ferdinand RF, Kasius MC. The prevalence of DSM-III-R diagnosis in a national sample of Dutch adolescents. *Archives of General Psychiatry* 1997;**54**:329–36.
3 Muris P, Meesters C, Merckelbach H, Sermon A, Zwakhalen S. Worry in normal children. *Journal of the American Academy of Child and Adolescent Psychiatry* 1998;**37**:703–10.
4 Silverman WK, Rabian B. Simple phobias. *Child and Adolescent Psychiatry Clinics of North America* 1993;**2**:603–23.
5 Klykylo WM, Kay J, Rube D. *Clinical child psychiatry*. Philadelphia: WB Saunders, 1998.
6 Last CG, Perrin S, Hersen M, Kazdin AE. DSM-III-R anxiety disorders in children: sociodemographic and clinical characteristics. *Journal of the American Academy of Child and Adolescent Psychiatry* 1992;**31**:1070–6.
7 Weiner IB. *Child and adolescent psychopathology*. New York: Wiley, 1982.
8 Macaulay JL, Kleinknecht RA. Panic and panic attacks in adolescents. *Journal of Anxiety Disorders* 1989;**3**:221–41.

Further reading

AACAP Official Action. Practice Parameters for the Assessment and Treatment of Children and Adolescents with Anxiety Disorders. *Journal of the American Academy of Child Psychology and Psychiatry* 1997;**36**:69S–84S.
King N, Tinge BJ, Heyne D *et al.* Cognitive-behavioral treatment of school refusing children: a controlled evaluation. *Journal of the American Academy of Child Psychology and Psychiatry* 1998;**37**:4395–403.

4: Post-traumatic stress disorder

Introduction

Post-traumatic stress disorder (PTSD) is a relatively recently recognised condition although it has probably long been in existence. It was first officially recognised as a syndrome in the 1980s and was grouped with the anxiety disorders. Three main constellations of symptoms were described:

- Distressing and recurring recollections of the trauma
- Avoidance of stimuli associated with the trauma
- Increased physiological arousal.

In day to day practice clinicians are most likely to see PTSD following abuse, life-threatening illness, or road traffic accidents. It is normal for children to respond to trauma with distress. However once the danger has passed such children should slowly return to normal. In PTSD the symptoms persist with intrusive images of the event as if they are re-experiencing it, or there is marked avoidance behaviour or significant physiological arousal.

Much of the literature is based on adults but it is likely that there will be more descriptions of PTSD in childhood in the near future.

Epidemiology

Many studies have shown that PTSD occurs in children from diverse ethnic and cultural backgrounds though the presentation may differ. The lifetime prevalence of PTSD has been reported to range between 1% and 14%. High risk groups include those exposed to community violence, life-threatening illness, or multiple stressors. Parental distress and/or parental psychiatric pathology increase the risk, while good family support and the ability of parents to cope with the trauma act as protecting factors.

Aetiology

Adult studies have suggested that there may be a genetic vulnerability to the development of PTSD, while three factors may mediate the development of PTSD in children:

- The severity of the trauma
- Trauma related parental distress
- Temporal proximity to the traumatic event.

Clinical presentation

The developmental stage of the child affects the clinical presentation, so that with increasing age, the presentation will resemble more closely the constellation of symptoms described in adults. Preschool children may present with generalised anxiety, sleeping difficulties, unfocused aggression, repetitive play about the trauma, avoidance of, or preoccupation with, specific situations, people or events. Similar symptoms may occur in school aged children, but avoidance, numbing and flashbacks are more likely than in the preschool group.

Children may avoid discussing their feelings with parents in order to minimise their own and their parents' distress. Adolescent survivors have an increased rate of depression, panic attacks, aggression, substance abuse, and self-injurious thoughts and behaviour. When the trauma has been recurrent such as often occurs with any form of abuse, there may be more symptoms of a dissociative nature.

Comorbidity

Associated problems include anxiety, depression, somatization, and conduct disorder.

Differential diagnosis

Much of what follows might be dismissed as pedantry. Without major classification schemes to guide or distract us we might not be too preoccupied with the differential diagnosis. However the first two conditions described below might be confused with PTSD.

Adjustment disorder

The symptoms occur after a trauma, but do not meet the full criteria for the diagnosis of PTSD. Such disorders if handled appropriately are self-limiting.

Acute stress disorder

The fundamental distinguishing factor between acute stress disorder and PTSD is that acute stress disorder occurs and resolves within 4 weeks of the traumatic event and lasts for a minimum of 2 days. If symptoms persist beyond 1 month however, then the diagnosis should be changed to PTSD.

Anxiety and depression

Affective symptoms such as anxiety (see chapter 3) and depression (see chapter 6) are common in general, and particularly so after a trauma. They may be comorbid with PTSD or primary.

Obsessive compulsive disorder

In obsessive compulsive disorder (see chapter 9) patients experience intrusive thoughts, but these are not related to a traumatic event. Generally they are considered inappropriate and are not associated with a feeling of actually reliving the event, as in flashbacks, or with a feeling of dissociation.

Psychotic disorder

Flashbacks may be confused with hallucinations, illusions or other perceptual disturbances that occur in some psychotic disorders (see chapter 12).

Treatment

In practice this involves a combination of parental counselling, cognitive behaviour therapy (see chapter 24), and medication for symptomatic relief (see chapter 25). There is very limited evidence to support the use of any medications specifically for PTSD.

A number of other treatments are being used and are worthy of consideration, and some of these are discussed below.

Eye movement desensitisation and reprocessing (EMDR)

This is an intervention that has been used in the adult population and has been shown clinically to be useful also in children. Full trials are awaited. It involves inducing eye movements while exposing the individual to intrusive thoughts of the trauma. The reasons for its apparent effectiveness are not yet understood.

Self help

A series of booklets for children suffering from the consequences of road traffic accidents and their carers have been produced. The books describe some of the possible reactions that the child may experience following the accident. It may be appropriate to routinely provide such information following an accident.

Group therapy

In traumatic situations which involve whole communities support groups are commonly used and perceived to be helpful. The groups allow the sharing of the emotional response as well as ways of solving common problems, thus facilitating a sense of mastery.

Prognosis

There have been few studies of the natural course of PTSD in children or of its treatments. What evidence there is suggests that prognosis varies from spontaneous remission through to chronicity.

Conclusion

A number of different types of severe life events can lead to the development of PTSD in children but the presentation may vary according to the developmental stage of the child, and the nature and longevity of the stress. Treatment is complex and is best provided within specialist services. The prognosis is variable.

Further reading

AACAP Official Action. Practice Parameters for the Assessment of Treatment of Children and Adolescents with Post-Traumatic Stress Disorder. *Journal of the American Academy of Child and Adolescent Psychiatry* 1998;**37**:4S–26S.

Child Accident Prevention Trust. *Getting over an accident.* London: Child Accident Prevention Trust, 1998.

Cohen J. Summary of the practice parameters for the assessment and treatment of children and adolescents with post-traumatic stress disorder. *Journal of the American Academy of Child and Adolescent Psychiatry* 1998; **37**:997–1001.

Foy DW, Madvig BT, Pynoos RS, Camilleri AJ. Etiologic factors in the development of post-traumatic stress disorders in children and adolescence. *Journal of School Psychology* 1996;**34**:133–45.

Yule W. Post-traumatic stress disorder. *Archives of Disease in Childhood* 1999;**80**:107–9.

5: The disruptive disorders

Introduction

Some children are troubled but do not trouble others except by way of inducing empathy with their distress. These children were once referred to as "neurotic" or having emotional disorders, and more recently internalizing disorders. They are more troubled than troubling to others. Some children trouble others but do not seem, and may not be, troubled themselves. These children were once referred to as having conduct disorders and more recently externalising disorders. The dominant feature of their presentation is disruption to others and to the course of their own lives rather than distress. In practice, most of those we see present mixed features of distress and disruption. They are both troubled and troubling. This chapter concentrates on those who mainly trouble others but who may also, at least partially and less obviously, be troubled within.

- Normal children can be "naughty" and we usually deal with naughtiness in normal children by being disapproving, angry, or withdrawing positive experiences.
- We may "punish" them in some way by providing negative consequences for the "naughtiness".
- "Naughtiness" normally involves doing things which:

  - Are unsafe or might risk danger to the child themselves, others, or valued possessions and property
  - Cause conflict with, or loss of respect from, others
  - Break down the usual cooperative rules that make daily life work more easily.

- However, there are times when "naughtiness" lasts longer, is more severe and has more negative consequences than is usual with most children.
- When disapproval, anger, withdrawal of positive experiences, and punishment do not work, we are increasingly likely to find a "moral framework" for understanding these children less helpful. We are likely then to use the concept of a disruptive disorder and approach the problem as a disorder to be treated rather than a failing or "sin" to be punished.

- Disruptive disorders disrupt the lives of others but the children's lives are also disrupted. Their mood may be anxious or depressed as their disorder persists. Their education will almost always suffer. Their self-esteem is slowly eroded. Their family life and friendships are steadily more conflicted. Their futures are less optimal than the children around them. A disproportionate number will find themselves in trouble with the law, out of a job and with failed relationships and marriages when they move into adulthood.

Aetiology

Where concentration and hyperactivity predominate (attention deficit hyperactivity disorder, ADHD) the causes are likely to be mainly genetic and to a smaller extent developmental and perinatal. When antisocial behaviour and conduct disorder predominate and concentration is intact (conduct disorder and oppositional disorder), environmental factors predominate. These include parents who are critical and chaotic, with discordant marriages or antisocial or criminal lifestyles. In practice these factors overlap. Children with ADHD, untreated, are likely to become increasingly oppositional and conduct disordered as they find themselves unable to meet the expectations for the behaviour demanded of them. Children who are initially oppositional within the home, and who remain untreated, are increasingly likely to generalise their behaviour to the school and to become oppositional to society as well as their parents, i.e. develop a conduct disorder. Only a minority (about one third) will go on to be antisocial in adulthood. However, this third are a very troubled and troubling minority who will preoccupy the lives of the families and friends of those close to them, the police, the courts, and society generally.

Clinical presentation

Overactivity

Parents and teachers vary in what they regard as an overactive child. If a child is overactive in most settings and there is a consensus that the child is more active than most other children, they are likely to be diagnosed with ADHD. They are even more likely to attract this diagnosis if their behaviour is less purposeful, less predictable, and more chaotic, and if they fail to persist with tasks or activities of interest to them. If they sleep less, seem to be oblivious to instruction, danger, and punishment, they will almost certainly be seen as having ADHD or the more serious hyperkinetic syndrome (hyperactive, impulsive, distractible and excitable behaviour which is pervasive in all settings). Occasionally, a child will have all these features together with not perceiving aspects of their environment which may lead to being injured, sometimes seriously. This is referred to as DAMP syndrome. That is they have deficits in attention, motor control, and perception. This is often associated with developmental difficulties and problems with understanding the emotions of others.

Concentration difficulties

Concentration is fundamental to learning certain abilities:

- To attend to what is happening around us
- To focus on what we need to do
- To follow through with a job, activity, project or task and to complete it
- To shift to the next task
- To sequence our tasks and activities.

Inability to do these things is often equated with disobedience, defiance, and failure.

Lack of cooperation

Learning to work together is vital for survival in a complex society. The most basic levels of cooperation are:

- Self-care and hygiene
- Sharing
- Learning for future survival and success
- Maintaining a friendship group
- Respecting the personal space and property rights of others.

Children with disruptive disorders are likely to have difficulties in each of these areas. Refusal to cooperate may involve fear of failure, anticipation of criticism, inability to show compassion for others, and lack of basic social skills and problem solving. Being exploitative or being exploited go together. The demanding, tyrannical young teenager who then goes out and is a "stooge" for a group's outrageous antisocial escapades highlights this strange mixture of non-cooperation and inappropriate cooperation—trusting antisocial peers and being wary of supportive adults.

Conflict and aggression

Refusal to cooperate, defiance and stubbornness can lead to a battle of wills between parent and child, teacher and child, or child with child. Conflict can arise for many other reasons, but the most common of these are:

- Parental anxieties about the child and the child's desire for freedom
- The child's fear of disapproval leading to angry, uncontrollable outbursts—temper tantrums
- The desire for retaliation on the part of a child, parent or sibling and the counter-retaliation
- Response to high levels of parental discord, conflict, anger, or aggression
- Maltreatment in the form of emotional, physical or sexual abuse.

Children usually test their capacities to disagree within the home. They hold to their own position and fend off demands for submission from others. Siblings practise dominance within the relative safety of parental arbitration. Usually, muted versions of sibling conflict also occur within the school context, again with the less reliably present oversight of a teacher during playground duty. However, in each of these situations, both at home and at school, some children will stand out as being more prone to conflict and aggression and less capable of social cooperation and reconciliation skills. "Bullies" and "victims" emerge, especially in a culture where "bully" teachers are tolerated and punitive disciplinary structures exist. Verbal disagreement and threat, physical pushing, shoving, holding, hurting and hitting are all common. Staring, glowering, raised voices, physical intimidation are all associated with dominance behaviour which is often impulsive. Planned predatory and secretive attacks are less common, more sinister in their long term significance and more likely to be associated with a criminal subculture. They are also less likely to be responsive to psychopharmacological and psychological treatment strategies.

Lying and stealing

As with all behaviours associated with breaking social rules, those committed within a group or as part of group activities are different from those committed as isolated individuals.

When lying and stealing usually reduces the harmful consequences of actions or increases the likelihood of a positive reward, they are likely to persist and become more expert. The more intelligent, socially experienced and otherwise friendly a young person is the more likely is their lying to be believed and the stealing to go undetected. For many children lying is their chief mechanism for avoiding abuse, exploiting a short term situation to their advantage, or exacting revenge on a rival. Stealing is their way of getting what they do not believe will come to them legitimately or has been withheld from them "unfairly". Children with long term resentment at "missing out" are very prone to steal. These symptoms are common in all disruptive disorders but especially the conduct disorders (see below).

Fire setting and vandalism

These are usually done secretly and in groups but occasionally they are solitary activities. The most worrying are the solitary, unprovoked and premeditated episodes. If either of these pictures occur "out of the blue" with no past history of behaviour difficulty or psychiatric disorder, then major depression, emerging psychosis or rarely an organic disorder need to be considered. Where they are not out of the blue they most usually are due to conduct disorders.

Where group fire setting and vandalism occur, urgent community consultation needs to occur to dismantle the group and provide strong positive alternative activities.

Truancy and running away from home

Running away from school or home are more common in those from antisocial, abusive or chaotic backgrounds. Characteristically such children are impulsive and traumatised. However, the teenager who runs away from home or school with little previous history of conduct problems or psychiatric disorder needs to be registered by all as a possible victim of abuse or suffering from a major psychiatric disorder in evolution. Late onset conduct disorder does occur, especially with adverse peer influence. However, there is a disproportionate number of these young people with affective and early schizophreniform disorders.

Three patterns of disruptive troubles

1. *Oppositional defiant disorder (ODD).* Those who struggle with those they love and with whom they live.
2. *Attention deficit disorder with or without hyperactivity (ADD and ADHD).* Those who struggle to control themselves and to maintain a focus.
3. *Conduct disorder (CD).* Those who struggle with most of the people they know and against society and its rules.

How do these patterns of disorder relate to one another?

The bulk of evidence suggests that ODD and CD are environmentally determined while ADHD has a large genetic contribution.

Marital discord, parental criticism, coercive parenting and chaotic family life contribute to ODD and CD. However ODD represents an earlier, milder and more circumscribed disorder. CD is the fully developed disruptive disorder. The more that disruptive behaviour is restricted to struggling with particular adults and the more discrepant that behaviour is between home and school, the more likely the disorder is to be ODD. The more the behaviour is generalised to different contexts, the more the struggle is against any adult and anyone (authority or otherwise) who thwarts, then the more likely is

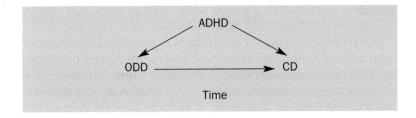

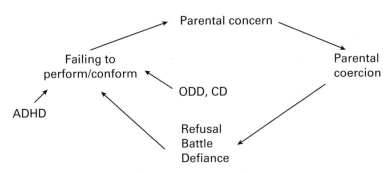

Figure 5.1   The concern–coercion cycle

the diagnosis to be CD. ADHD predisposes to ODD when parents try to push children with ADHD to cooperate and to perform. The children respond by struggling, failing, resisting, and defying (Figure 5.1).

The double life of the ODD child

Many children with early ODD may be struggling and battling with parents at home while being well behaved at school or other people's homes. These children are sometimes described as "indoor devils and outdoor saints". Parents may be particularly hurt and angry that their opposition is reserved for them alone. Strangely there is sometimes a relief when parents find others are beginning to have difficulties with their children even though it clearly bodes ill for the child. In the parents' minds it confirms that their child is generally difficult.

ADHD

ADHD is not a single condition but a variety of conditions with a final common pathway of clinical presentation. There are also many other conditions that may result in impairment of attention, for example head injury, intellectual impairment, frontal lobe damage, psychosis, severe anxiety and depression. Each may require very different treatments.

ADHD is a diagnosis that is capable of being overdiagnosed because many of the behaviours are common in the normal population when children are excited, tired, overstimulated, frustrated, or poorly supervised.

There is a high genetic contribution to the picture. It is not surprising therefore that many of the parents are excitable, chaotic, distractible and at times inattentive, i.e. the parents may have part of the spectrum of behaviours associated with ADHD. This partly explains why many therapists are convinced that ADHD is the outcome of poor parenting.

Highly motivated parents are likely to overemphasise ADHD in dreamy, academically underperforming teens. Those less well informed and resourced may overlook true cases of ADHD because they are not hyperactive. Different families will have different thresholds for what is judged overactive. However children who are judged persistently overactive by parents, teachers and an experienced clinician are likely to have true ADHD and to respond to pharmacological treatment.

CD

Behaviour which is defiant of adults and undertaken despite adult censure might be termed conduct disorder. It might alternatively be framed individualism, determination, or strength of character. However, the term conduct disorder is normally reserved for well established uncooperative and antisocial behaviour which has a marked negative impact on the child's life, educational achievement, and friendships. In general, the earlier the onset, the longer the duration, the more solitary the activities, the more interlocked with a criminal environment and the more severe the behaviours, the more likely is the disorder to persist into adulthood.

Tips for assessing the child with conduct disorder are given in Box 5.1.

Box 5.1 Five tips in assessing the child with conduct disorder

1. The diagnosis should not be made on a cross-sectional picture only. The longitudinal history may be essential. For example, a history of CD after a head injury may reflect frontal lobe damage. An adolescent onset CD may reflect an emerging psychosis. Sudden onset CD in a primary school age child may bespeak abuse or an intolerable family situation
2. Target comorbidity wherever possible. Anxiety, depression, post-traumatic stress disorder, ADHD and any other comorbid conditions should be considered. Medical comorbidity must also be considered. Any condition which compromises frontal inhibition of inappropriate social behaviour should be considered
3. Substance abuse causes CD as well as resulting from it. Short term experimentation, self-medication for dysphoria and peer related group substance abuse may all give rise to a picture that in a different context would have a more grave significance
4. The same phenomena in adolescence may have a significantly better prognosis than when seen in adulthood. It is imperative not to assess phenomena in isolation from the life stage in which they occur. This is not an argument for complacency in adolescence but against nihilism in CD
5. Avoid trying to treat CD by disapproval. CD is a description not an explanation. Assumptions which involve parental failure, character inadequacy, deliberate wickedness and the need for moral awakening may all be important in society as a whole but are relatively unhelpful for the practical clinician who wishes to proceed beyond a strategic "tut tut"

Treatment

ODD

Support the carer(s)

Avoid being critical of critical parents. It often makes them more critical. Identifying positive aspects of parenting is likely to encourage improvements in parenting. Of course there are times when such strategies are unsuccessful, but the benefit of the doubt towards the parent is the most helpful initial approach.

Identify the child in whom reliance is a major issue as well as defiance

Parents who find themselves doing everything and being increasingly criticised the more they do need to appreciate the degree of reliance their child has upon them. The defiance can then be framed in the context of the child protesting against being treated as a younger child but also reluctant to assume the responsibilities of a more mature child. Incremental promotion of greater responsibility with definitely manageable goals gradually reverses this negative cycle.

Point out the unhelpful cycles of interaction to everyone in the family

Identifying the specifics of negative cycles of interaction, together with positive alternatives, can be very helpful for both parents and children. This needs to be done sympathetically and with the awareness that most people do not try to be negative or to create negative cycles. Just making explicit these patterns of negative interaction can change behaviour. Paradoxically, reassuring parents and children that they should not try to change everything at once and that many of these cycles take many months to change frees the family not to get too disappointed about the pace of change.

Encourage the children to see their own good points

Most children with disruptive disorders no longer hear positive comments about themselves or see a positive future for themselves. Help the parents to do this without appearing to be naïve to the difficulties they have faced as parents. Focussed work on the child's self-esteem is essential.

Develop a plan of educational assessment and management with the school

Identify any learning difficulties, and areas of strength and weakness, so that a long term plan can be implemented across school and home.

Try to reduce secondary complications

When the family members feel shame, anxiety and depression about their difficulties, these sometimes need to be addressed directly. Weariness, despair and the desperate search for "make or break" solutions are common. The competent clinician who communicates respect for patients and their parents will reduce these complications.

ADHD

Normalising naughtiness

Educating parents and those responsible for children's care about ADHD means communicating some of these simple themes:

- ADHD is not naughtiness
- All naughtiness is not due to ADHD
- Children with ADHD can still be naughty
- Normal children sometimes have concentration difficulties.

Stimulation, structure, and supervision

Try always to have something for them to do but not so much so as to overwhelm the child: all children have a stimulus window. If they are understimulated they will become bored and misbehave. If they are overstimulated they will become overwhelmed and misbehave. Children with ADHD and other neurodevelopmental problems have narrowed stimulus windows, i.e. they become both understimulated and overstimulated more easily than normal children. They always need something to do but never too much. They are worse in supermarkets, crowds and at parties because of overstimulation. They misbehave or get into difficulties when left on their own, unsupervised and without something specific to do which falls within their skill range.

Education at school

Such children benefit from being in smaller classes, with less distraction, and low intensity teachers who are not easily upset and who focus on:

- The interests of the children
- Well graduated learning increments
- Visual, activity based work rather than verbal and written work alone
- Rewards for persistence and patience, albeit fleeting at times.

The possibility of repeating an academic year might be considered.

Medication

- *Stimulants.* The evidence for the use of stimulants for the treatment of concentration difficulties and the associated behavioural difficulties is overwhelming, with more than a hundred double blind randomised controlled trials. Despite the controversy surrounding their usage, they are the psychotropics with the longest history of usage and one of the lowest profiles of adverse effect. Methylphenidate and dexamfetamine are the two main stimulants (see chapter 25 for dosage details).
- *Amitriptyline.* This also has been demonstrated to be a helpful medication for attentional difficulties. It has the added advantages of helping with anxiety, insomnia, and enuresis. It is best used as a second-line medication.
- *Clonidine.* This medication has weak evidence for its efficacy and generally has very few side effects. It also helps with sleep, anxiety and is said to be better with angry, impulsive children. There is little solid evidence on this. It does have one very serious drawback. If children or their parents withdraw the drug abruptly it can cause rebound hypertension, i.e. high blood pressure, which can be life threatening.

Parental support and education

Encouraging parents to look after themselves and recruiting extended family, friends and others to provide respite are all important. The single biggest difficulty is secondary behavioural complications leading to oppositional behaviour and conduct disorder. Avoiding coercive parenting styles and encouraging clear expectations with support and comfort rather than criticism are essential. "Supporting the child doing the right thing" and letting the child know when he or she has done the right thing must slowly replace the tendency to nag and harp about inadequacy, incompetency, and doing the wrong thing.

Self-esteem

As with ODD enhancing the child's self-esteem is an essential part of the treatment programme, given that such children are so used to being criticised and blamed.

Conclusion

ADHD is a real syndrome of disability buried in an epidemic of overdiagnosis on the one hand and the outraged denials of its existence on the other. It is strongly genetic, generally treatment responsive, but highly damaging to educational progress and self esteem if left untreated. There is a high comorbidity with learning disorder and secondary oppositional and conduct disorder. Anxiety and depression are frequently associated. There is increasing evidence that there are different varieties of ADHD with different underlying brain difficulties.

Conduct disorder

Everything that has been written about both ODD and ADHD is applicable to conduct disorder. However, several further issues should be emphasised.

Keep parental expectations of change low

Conduct disorder is a chronic disorder with potentially serious complications. It is best to work on a sympathetic but palliative model with the possibility of occasional surprises.

Keep long term expectations
for a better outcome modestly high

Our capacity to predict is sufficiently inaccurate to encourage everyone dealing with antisocial young people to remain modestly optimistic. For most parents, especially early on in these disorders, gentle and modest optimism is helpful.

When disappointments are frequent

There may be a time when it helps the parents and siblings to manage and be more sympathetic if they despair of a child's capacity to change. Reducing expectations reduces frustration and disappointment. If this can be achieved without rejection it may occasionally produce positive change.

Self-esteem

As with ODD and ADHD, enhancing the child's self-esteem is crucial. Despite any apparent bravado, such children usually have poor self-esteem which exacerbates the behavioural difficulties.

Treatment of comorbidity

This should always be incorporated even when there is despair about affecting the core disruptive behaviour.

Prognosis

ODD has an increasing likelihood of becoming CD if it persists beyond 8 years of age. Untreated ADHD is likely to be complicated by CD and may persist into adulthood with a range of disorders. CD has a strong continuity into adult years with a personality disorder commonly developing. There is a disturbingly high rate of accident and death in the disruptive disorders especially CD. However, despite discouraging legacies there is a significant minority who do well. Prognostic humility demands that we keep an open mind wherever possible even if our mode of care is palliative in nature.

Conclusion

There has been much more interest in the disruptive disorders in recent years. Treatments are still less than satisfactory. Although there are a number of preventive and early intervention programmes, most are not geared for the busy clinician over brief time intervals. Most medication interventions focus on concentration difficulties although conduct disorders are known to benefit as well. Particular attention should be paid to supporting the parents and enhancing the child's self-esteem. The prognosis remains guarded and sometimes clearly negative, but a significant minority of these patients do well.

Further reading

Gilberg C (1995) *Clinical child neuropsychiatry*. Cambridge: Cambridge University Press, 2001.

Hill J, Maughan B, eds. *Conduct disorders in childhood and adolescence*. Cambridge: Cambridge University Press, 2001.

MTA Cooperative Group. A 14 month randomised controlled trial of treatment strategies for attention deficit/hyperactivity disorder. *Archives of General Psychiatry* 1999;56:1073–86.

Smith DJ. Youth crime and conduct disorder: trends patterns and causal explanations. In: Rutter M, Smith DJ, eds. *Psychosocial disorders in young people—time trends and their causes*. Chichester: Wiley, 1995.

6: Depression and suicidality

Introduction

Depression in childhood was once thought to be rare, short lived, relatively harmless, and responsive to even minor intervention. It is now clear that childhood and adolescent depression has the potential for being a serious illness that is far more common and potentially damaging than previously realised.

Definition

Depression can be:

- A symptom: for example, "he seems depressed", "I feel depressed"
- A syndrome: i.e. a cluster of symptoms such as marked sadness, tearfulness, and loss of appetite
- A disorder: i.e. a specific disorder fulfilling diagnostic criteria (see below) of which there are different types.

In childhood and adolescence it is debatable how useful it is to attempt to distinguish between these concepts and indeed between the different types of depression. It is probably more useful to conceptualise depression along a continuum. At the mild end would be occasional feelings of sadness or misery and at the severe end would be suicidal despair or complete and persistent psychomotor retardation. What is most important is how the problem is managed. The more the child is suffering the more important it is to offer appropriate treatment, regardless of whether what is presented is a symptom, a syndrome, or a disorder. The nature and severity of depression in the younger population is determined to some extent by developmental considerations.

Developmental considerations

In the face of inescapable adversity children may become immobile, passive, unresponsive, and helpless at any age.

Preschool children may look miserable and cry on a sustained basis in the face of abandonment, social disruption, or trauma. They may have altered sleep, appetite and psychomotor mobility, but few can consistently articulate their feelings. From the age of about 6 children begin to identify and verbalise feelings of sadness. Between 7 and 8 they have the ability for sustained beliefs about themselves, including negative beliefs. In later childhood and adolescence this ability may extend to negative views and generalizations about any aspect of life.

Epidemiology

At any one time between 0·5% and 2·5% of preadolescents and 2% and 8% of adolescents will be suffering from depression. It occurs more frequently in older adolescents (15–19 years) with a female preponderance in adolescents but not preadolescents. Children living in a socially and economically deprived environment are at higher risk.

Aetiology

Risk factors for depression include:

- *Age.* Depression increases after puberty until the mid twenties.
- *Gender.* In the prepubertal child the sex ratio is equal, but in adolescence there is a female preponderance as seen in the adult population.
- *Family history.* Children with a parent or sibling suffering from depression or bipolar disorder have up to 10 times the risk of the normal population of developing such a disorder. There is also an increased risk following loss of a parent.
- *Family dysfunction.* Any form of family dysfunction, for example marital disharmony, may predispose to depression.
- *Past history of depression.* Many children relapse over time. However the outcome is far better for those who are treated with antidepressants for at least 6 months. Earlier cessation of treatment worsens the prognosis.
- *Serious academic problems.* Learning difficulties predispose to lowered mood.

- *Substance abuse.* This may occur as a consequence of depression or as a result; a significant minority are trapped in a self-defeating cycle where dysphoria causes craving but the substance gives little relief and sets the scene for further craving.
- *Anxiety disorders.* Chronic anxiety often leads to depression.
- *Abuse.* There is a higher rate of anxiety, depression, hopelessness and suicide in those who have been abused.
- *Medical conditions.* Any medical condition may predispose to depression, especially when chronic, severe or life threatening.
- *Vulnerable temperament.* Poor self-esteem, emotional sensitivity, a negative thinking style, and poor social skills may all predispose to depression.
- *Life events* such as bereavement and physical illness precede many depressive episodes.

Clinical features

Most of life is fraught with fluctuations in mood and childhood is no exception. Many children will feel sad and miserable on occasions but would not be considered to be depressed. A "rule of three" might be useful here. A child may have all the symptoms of depression for 3 days but it would not be useful to label this depression unless it is so extreme as to endanger safety. However, as sadness and suffering persists, becomes more severe, and affects many areas of life, the likelihood of this being a depressive syndrome or disorder requiring a professional response increases. After 3 days consideration should be given to the fact that this may be a persistent problem. After 3 weeks professional help is clearly needed. At 3 months the problem is established and by 3 years depression is well and truly long term. These time frames are conservative. Despite this, children and adolescents are often left for much longer periods in the belief that they will "self-correct", or "grow out of it", or that their suffering cannot be that bad because they are "only children".

The following features are indicative of a depressive disorder:

- Sad mood or loss of interest or pleasure.
- Irritability.

- Loss of weight, marked change in sleep pattern, loss of appetite.
- Psychomotor agitation or retardation (inability to sit still, temper tantrums or inability to get started are characteristic).
- Reduction in energy levels, fatigue, and boredom.
- Feelings of worthlessness or guilt (in children and young people this is usually attributed to what others think of them).
- Impaired thinking, concentration or decision making with deterioration in schoolwork and school refusal. This is among the most frequent problems and the most overlooked or attributed to other factors such as motivation, disinterest, or just plain "scatty".
- Anhedonia (an inability to enjoy pleasurable activities).
- Social withdrawal.
- Combativeness with parents.
- Loss of interest in schoolwork.
- Delinquent behaviour.
- Recurrent thoughts of death or suicide.

Depression may also occur comorbid to eating disorders (see chapter 8) and disruptive disorders (see chapter 5).

Psychotic depression

Any of the above features may be accompanied by an apparent loss of contact with reality. Delusions or hallucinations, with a depressive and self-critical or self-punitive content, are prominent. Such a picture is sometimes described as psychotic depression.

Bipolar disorder

Occasionally children present with what may appear to be the opposite to depression—mood elevation and lability, excitability, irritability, excess energy, lack of judgement, and disinhibition. Such states are known as hypomania and may occur alone or may alternate with episodes of depression. When mania occurs with no history of depression, or vice versa depression occurs with no history of mania, this is known as a unipolar disorder. When both occur either within the same time frame or quite distinctly, this is known as a bipolar disorder.

Suicidal behaviour

Any depressed child or adolescent is at risk of suicidal behaviour. Although rare before puberty, suicide is second only to accidental death in adolescence in several countries.

Suicide rates increase with age, with females more commonly dying of overdose and males from such methods as hanging, carbon monoxide poisoning, and shooting. For every fatality there are at least 100 attempts. In the USA up to 2% of high school students have made suicide attempts that have come to medical attention, with larger numbers making less serious attempts. Completed suicide occurs in about 1/100 000 preadolescents and 13/100 000 adolescents, with boys exceeding girls by 4 to 1.

Risk factors for completed suicide and suicide attempts

These risk factors are summarised in Table 6.1. It is clear that there are no definite discriminators of risk between attempters and completers. Being an attempter is one of the best predictors of likely completion. Suicidal behaviour should never be taken lightly. Warning signs are given in Box 6.1.

Differential diagnosis in the depressed child

This includes:

- Normal reactive feelings of sadness
- Anorexia nervosa
- Severe anxiety
- Disruptive disorder
- ADHD.

Table 6.1 Risk factors for completed suicide and suicide attempts

Suicidal ideation and/or attempts	Completed suicide
Females Previous suicide attempt and ideation	Males Previous suicide attempt and ideation
Major or minor depressive disorder	Familial psychiatric disorder and completed suicide attempt. Mood disorder—60%
Substance abuse Antisocial behaviour	Alcohol or drug abuse (particularly in males) Antisocial behaviour
Undesirable life events	Acute life crisis
Problems with parents, partners, school, or work	Disciplinary crisis/dispute with friend or parent
Loss in males Sexual or physical abuse	Legal or disciplinary problems in past year
	Availability of lethal arms, for example firearms in the home

Modified from Williams K. Preventing suicide in young people: what is known and what is needed. *Child: Care, Health and Development* 1997;**23**:173–85.

- Medical disorders such as epilepsy, systemic lupus erythematosus, traumatic brain injury, space occupying lesion, endocrinopathies, and dementias
- Adverse drug reactions, for example clonidine, stimulants and steroids
- Substance abuse (in particular ecstasy, amphetamines, barbiturates, and cocaine)
- Psychosis.

Assessment of suicidal ideation and behaviour

A detailed and skilled psychological assessment is mandatory. Asking about suicidal thoughts in young people who are at risk will not encourage suicidal behaviour. On the contrary, it would be dangerous to manage such situations without knowing of any suicidal thinking.

Box 6.1 Warning signs for suicide behaviour

In the short term:

- Thoughts of suicide as a solution to a problem
- References to suicide in conversation, for example "you will not need to worry about me for much longer"
- Disciplinary crisis or expulsion from school
- Preparation in the form of writing a will or a final message, or acquisition of means
- Increase in help seeking behaviour—about half of those making suicide attempts will have seen a doctor in the preceding month and a quarter within a week of the attempt
- Improvement of mood directly beforehand; a feeling of resolution may replace the feeling of distress once the decision to die has been made
- During the early stages of treatment the patient is particularly vulnerable to suicide. Improved psychomotor function from medication with increased energy and thoughts may precede improvement in mood and distress, and so lead to a suicidal attempt
- Recurrence of a situation that preceded a previous attempt of self-harm

In the longer term:

- Psychiatric morbidity (90% of completed suicides have a pre-existing psychiatric disorder), in particular depression, substance abuse disorders, and disruptive disorders
- Previous suicide attempts of patient or parent especially when accompanied by a strong desire to die
- Recent losses
- Hopelessness
- Lack of confiding friend and isolation
- Learning disorder or academic underachievement
- History of violent or impulsive behaviour
- Social disadvantage: broken home, unwanted pregnancy, conflict with parents, sexual, and physical or emotional abuse. Sexually abused girls are 20 times more likely and sexually abused boys 40 times more likely to commit suicide

An adolescent who has attempted suicide but remains silent, refusing to confirm or deny such thoughts, should be considered suicidal until proven otherwise.

The assessment should include exploring suicidal ideation, intent and plans, and the documentation of any previous attempts.

Suicidal ideation

Questions that can be asked to elicit ideation include:

- Have you ever just wanted to get away from it all?
- Do you ever feel like going to sleep and not waking up?
- Have you ever wished that you could die?

If the child confirms any of the above thoughts, then their severity, frequency and persistence all need to be further explored.

Suicidal intent

Suggested questions covering content include:

- Have you ever wanted to hurt yourself?
- In what ways have you thought about hurting yourself?
- Do you want to hurt yourself now?
- Do you want to die now?

Suicidal plans

What plans have been made and their effectiveness need to be explored next:

- Has there been a warning or help seeking behaviour?
- What evidence of planning or premeditation has been made, for example a suicidal note, a will?
- How lethal/effectively would the means be, if implemented?
- How angry and disappointed is the child at having been found?
- Have they been resistant to treatment subsequently?

Previous attempts

Previous attempts, the degree of lethality, precipitating circumstances and consequences need to be explored. It must be remembered that a previous attempt is the best predictor of completed suicide.

Although not to be used instead of a full assessment, the PATHOS instrument,[1] illustrated in Box 6.2, may be a useful aid:

> ## Box 6.2 The PATHOS instrument[1]. NB: this is not to be used instead of full assessment
>
> (P) Have you had Problems for longer than 1 month?
> (A) Were you Alone in the house at the time?
> (T) Did you plan the overdose for longer than Three hours?
> (HO) Are you feeling HOpeless about the future?
> (S) Were you feeling Sad for most of the time before the overdose?
>
> Scale score is sum of questions:
> Score 1 for Yes; 0 for No. High risk group if score more than 2

Treatment

The key components of treatment include deciding on the most appropriate setting for treatment, engaging and educating the young person and family, cognitive behavioural therapy (see chapter 24), family therapy (see chapter 22), psychopharmacology (see chapter 25), residential treatment, and ECT. Liaison with the school is not only helpful in diagnosis but also creates a supportive environment for the child.

A treatment plan should be worked out, helping the adolescent to make suggestions about practical and achievable plans to improve the situation. "Contracts" and crisis plans with contact telephone numbers, can be used to encourage appropriate help seeking if feeling suicidal in the future. It is often surprising to clinicians that adolescents take contracts or "giving their word" so seriously. It should be remembered that some young people are prone to suicidal behaviour precisely because they have an overburdened sense of responsibility. This can be sometimes utilised to good effect.

In the depressed child parents should be told that it is a common disorder, with generally a good outcome, treatments on the whole are successful but take time and recurrence is high. The depression should be normalised without minimising, environmental stressors reduced, and access to means of self-harm removed.

In the child with bipolar disorder the family need to know:

- This is a serious disorder with grave outcome without treatment but a guardedly optimistic outcome with treatment.

- It is extremely difficult for the young person to have to live with such variable and, at times, unpredictable, emotions.
- Concentration, the ability to stay on task and make decisions are virtually impossible when mood is high.
- Even slight parental ambivalence about the value of medication is likely to result in poor adherence.
- This is a potentially lifelong disorder to which the whole family will need to make adjustments.

Encourage the child to avoid:

- Alcohol, illegal drugs, sleep deprivation, academic and work pressure, or pretending that nothing is wrong.

Encourage the parents to avoid:

- *Self-blame.* Parents need to be absolved of responsibility for the disorder even when there may be ways in which they could have been better parents. It is difficult for parents to believe, especially when their children are depressed, that they have done all they should have done.
- *Exhaustion.* Parents need to take care of themselves and the siblings of the affected child. Exhaustion, despair, unrealistic abiding expectations, fears of siblings being similarly affected may all oscillate like a pendulum with the patient.
- *Psychological cause hunting.* The overwhelming evidence is that psychoses are not caused by adverse life events or early relationship difficulties, though these may play a role in precipitating the illness or contributing to relapse.

The young person needs to know that:

- What they are experiencing is a serious disorder.
- If they are manic, then almost nothing will convince them they are unwell at that time unless there is associated desperation and agitation.
- When they are in a mixed state, confusion, fear and agitation should be linked to their illness.
- The more negative symptoms at any stage can be linked legitimately to illness, rather than to medication, the more likely are they to comply with treatment.
- They are grappling with one of the "malignancies" of psychiatry which, nevertheless does respond to treatment.

- They have to reduce their expectations when it comes to concentration.
- They and their families should avoid upsetting movies, books, friends or family members, large gatherings and long distance travels.
- They should not try to resolve longstanding interpersonal issues and make major decisions.
- The clinician's advice will often have much more importance than many clinicians realise. Giving advice that creates options rather than restricts, takes advantages of strengths rather than exposes weaknesses and follows premorbid trajectories rather than illness related enthusiasms or aversions, is essential wisdom for these disorders.
- When a lower mood is settling in it is often helpful to find something a little more active to do or a friend who lifts the spirits so that boredom and despair will not always be an inevitable progression.
- How to set a daily timetable which stops them from doing too much when they are elated or confused.
- The episodes last for several months and, even if medication abolishes symptoms, the episode is "going on" underneath. Mood stabilising medication yields better results the longer and more consistently it is used.
- When hope is lost, emphasise the phasic nature of this disorder and that when hope returns much that looks impossible now will happen as a matter of course.

Psychopharmacology

The first line drugs used are selective serotonin reuptake inhibitors (SSRIs; see chapter 25, for example fluoxetine); others used in clinical practice include sertraline, paroxetine and fluvoxamine, and the new reversible monoamine oxidase inhibitors (RIMAs). SSRIs are on the whole well tolerated and present minimal danger in overdose. If the child fails to respond to initial pharmacotherapy then consider the following:

- Increasing the dose of medication.
- Substituting with another mediaction.
- Augmenting the initial treatment.
- Using a combination of medications.

Second line medications include venlafaxine and nefazadone. Drugs that have been used for augmentation include lithium and thyroxine. Care needs to be taken when combining these drugs with an SSRI as they may cause the serotonin syndrome and alter drug levels of the drugs used. Thus it is best when drug augmentation or combination therapy is used, to proceed in liaison with a psychiatric colleague. The less experienced may feel the need to liaise at an earlier stage. However, with further experience confidence will grow by seeing children and young people respond to the practical management suggested here. Since the depressed are at an increased risk of suicide either appropriate supervision of medications by parents or guardians should be carried out or these drugs should be prescribed at times of high risk in a batch adequate to last for a week. Tricyclics are not recommended for the treatment of depression in this age group as they are less effective, have unpleasant side effects, and are dangerous in overdose.

The young person should be warned that these medications take 3 days to adjust to for initial side effects, 3 weeks for improvement in mood to begin to take place, and 3 months for the full benefit to be evident. They will need to stay on them for a minimum of 12 months since the evidence now suggests that if depression is treated earlier and more thoroughly, chronicity and recurrence are less likely.

Treating psychotic depression

It is wise to treat the prominent feature; if depression predominates use antidepressants, if psychosis predominates use newer antipsychotics such as risperidone or olanzapine.

The clinician should be aware of the potential for a shift into hypomania. The psychotic young person is at high risk of developing bipolar disorder.

Treating agitation

Among all the symptoms of psychotic depression, agitation is one of the most distressing. It is often difficult to distinguish akathisia (see chapter 25) from psychotic agitation.

Antipsychotics should be given until the symptoms of psychosis are controlled.

Minimise the impact of adverse reactions

It is important to take side effects seriously and make a decision as to what can be addressed immediately and what must wait until the young person improves. Weight gain on antipsychotics, nausea on SSRIs and mild oversedation on benzodiazepines all need to be addressed but may be tolerated in the acute phase. However, akathisia, unstable temperature or ataxia would all require immediate re-evaluation of medication and action. Idiosyncratic tolerance of side effects may need to be considered. Some boys may tolerate gross tremor but not loss of libido, and others vice versa.

Treating bipolar disorder

The first priority is to find an effective and tolerable medication regimen. In the depressive phase, antidepressants as described above are required. In the hypomanic phase sedation is indicated. Mood stabilisers such as lithium or carbamazepine should also be considered (see chapter 25).

Indications for hospitalisation

Hospitalisation should be considered for assessment of suicidal ideation or behaviour, poorly controlled depression or hypomania, or psychotic features.

ECT

This should only be considered for the very unresponsive depressed, psychotic or suicidal child. Up to two thirds of those under 18 years with resistant or psychotic depression improve. In severe cases ECT usually works faster and more effectively than medication with minimal longer term adverse effects. However, so effective has been the campaign in the public mind against ECT that it must be reserved till the last and many parents will refuse, fearing their child will be damaged by it. Applying an electrical impulse to the heart has, by way of contrast, been given a place of esteem in our medical treatments. As a result it will probably be some time before young people who have very severe depression will receive the same treatment options as adults.

Prognosis

Mild depression is often self-limiting although it may take up to several months to resolve. The more severe the depression the longer it takes to be treated and the more likelihood there is of relapse. Medication should be maintained for several months after apparent resolution to reduce the risk of relapse.

Conclusion

Depression is more common than is generally realised, may present in many different forms, and requires a comprehensive treatment approach. Early recognition and appropriate treatment are the best prognostic factors.

Psychotic depression and bipolar disorder are less common and require vigorous treatment. Suicidal ideation and behaviour should always be assessed and appropriate safeguards taken when present.

References

1 Kingsbury S. PATHOS: a screening instrument for adolescent overdose: a research note. *Journal of Child Psychology* 1996;37:609–11.

Further reading

Cochrane Database of Systemic Reviews. Fluoxetine decreased depressive symptoms in children and adolescents with nonpsychotic major depressive disorder. *Evidence-Based Medicine* 1998;3:105.

Kutcher SP. *Child and adolescent psychopharmacology.* Philadelphia: WB Saunders, 1997.

NHMRC. *Depression in young people. A guide for general practitioners.* National Health and Medical Research Council. Clinical Practice Guidelines. Canberra: Australian Government Publishing Service, 1997.

Reinecke MA, Ryan NE, DuBois DL. Cognitive-behavioural therapy of depression and depressive symptoms during adolescence: a review and meta-analysis. *Journal of the American Academy of Child and Adolescent Psychiatry* 1998;**37**:26–34.

Shaffer D, Fisher P, Dulcan MK, *et al.* The NIMH Diagnostic Interview Schedule for Children, version 2.3 (Disc–2.3): description, acceptability, prevalence rates and performance in the methods for the Epidemiology of Child and Adolescent Mental Disorders (MECA) study. *Journal of American Academy of Child and Adolescent Psychiatry* 1996;**35**:865–77.

Sprague T. Clinical management of suicidal behaviour in children and adolescents. *Clinical Child Psychology and Psychiatry* 1997:**2**:113–123.

Walter R. Half a century of ECT use in young people. *American Journal of Psychiatry* 1997;**154**:595–602.

7: Substance misuse

Introduction

Substance abuse is very common and capable of inducing almost any psychiatric disorder by altering the fundamental machinery of thought and emotion in the central and autonomic nervous systems. Alcohol and nicotine remain the most enjoyed and the most lethal. In general, public concern focuses on those substances that have:

- Immediate or short term medical threats
- Immediate socially adverse effects
- Appeal to the young
- A higher likelihood of producing psychotic phenomena
- Unpredictable behavioural effects
- Long lasting effects, especially cognitive and medical
- Ireversible effects
- A shorter track record with the public and therefore less familiarity.

Thus, nicotine remains a low risk in the public mind despite high long term morbidity and mortality, alcohol and marijuana a medium but familiar risk, and phencyclidine, heroin and lysergic acid, high risks. In absolute numbers of mortality, morbidity and burden of suffering these perceived risks are quite misleading. "Old demons" are less terrifying to the public consciousness even if they terrify more individuals and their families more often. Nicotine's legacy comes late and does not directly impair cognition. Its capacity to relax and reduce agitation override longer term considerations. Alcohol is so widely used as an anxiolytic and to facilitate socialisation that an inability to manage adverse effects is often put down to developmental immaturity or individual weakness. Similarly, the capacity of marijuana to induce psychosis is minimised by pointing out that these individuals were at risk anyway, that marijuana is much less toxic than alcohol, it grows naturally, and that it is helpful in chronic pain. It is very relaxing for many and reduces social anxiety in the short term. The main problems in dealing with substance use disorders is of providing effective, competing, less harmful alternative strategies for their perceived benefits and of helping cope with the difficulty of giving up.

Substance use disorders include both having difficulties with the impact of a particular substance and/or dependence on the substance itself.

Definitions

Substance abuse

The use of substances in a maladaptive manner causing mental, social or physical impairment.

Substance dependence

A constellation of symptoms with three or more of the following:

- Compulsion to take a substance
- Difficulties in controlling substance taking behaviour
- Physiological withdrawal state when substance not taken
- Evidence of tolerance (increasing doses required to achieve same effect)
- Progressive neglect of alternative pleasures or interests
- Persisting with substance use despite clear evidence of harmful consequences.

These criteria are based on adult classifications. Adolescents less frequently display withdrawal or symptoms of dependence but commonly exhibit tolerance, that is escalating doses required to get the same effect.

Epidemiology

Roughly 90% of students will have tried alcohol by the time they leave school, with approximately 30% of adolescent males reporting problem drinking. The American Association for Child and Adolescent Psychiatry has reported that around 40% will have tried an illicit drug, usually marijuana, with around 10% of 17–19 year olds having a lifetime prevalence of drug abuse or dependence. These figures are likely to be an underestimate.

Aetiology

Adolescent males predominate and comorbid disruptive disorder and mood disorders are frequent. Conduct disorder, attention deficit hyperactivity disorder, depression, social phobia, bulimia nervosa and post-traumatic stress disorder often precede and accompany substance use disorders. Panic and generalised anxiety disorder follow the substance misuse. Psychoses, both schizophreniform and mood related, are also important and need to be excluded as underlying causes. Psychoses are caused by substance abuse and predispose to substance abuse. The relationship is complex and in practice the busy clinician is often left managing a synergistic spiral of deteriorating function involving predisposing factors to mental illness and precipitating substance use.

Elements that increase an adolescent's risk include:

- *Familial factors* such as parental substance use, family dysfunction, and inadequate parenting.
- *Genetic vulnerability.* Alcohol abuse and dependence are both known to have strong genetic contributors. High novelty seeking and low harm avoidance have been identified as behavioural phenotypes of genetic vulnerability to substance use disorders.
- *Environmental factors* include peer pressure to use substances, low social economic status, increased crime, high population density, and ready availability of drugs.
- *Individual factors* include disruptive behaviour in early childhood, poor academic achievement, and risk taking behaviour.
- *Mental illness.* Any condition which increases impulsivity, anxiety and agitation and reduces judgement and mood level promotes substance misuse.
- *Gatekeeper or gateway substances.* There is evidence that some substances increase the likelihood of taking others,

for example nicotine may increase the likelihood of ingesting alcohol and vice versa, marijuana may increase the likelihood of taking amphetamines, alcohol may increase the likelihood of using MDMA ("ectasy"). The most important single adage is that most people are more likely to abuse two drugs if they abuse one. Coabuse and coaddiction are common.

Clinical features

Most substance-using adolescents use multiple substances (polysubstance abuse) and many will have coexisting psychiatric conditions. The substance-using adolescent may present with changes in behaviour, mood, and cognition. Behavioural changes include altered activity, disinhibition and hypervigilance—overactive, "over-the-top", and on guard. Cognitive disturbances include reduced attention and concentration, perceptual disturbances, and delusions. Changes in mood include euphoria, depression, and anxiety.

As a result the adolescent may display poor academic functioning and increased interpersonal conflict. The substance misuse may have adverse legal consequences such as being charged with possession of drugs, risk taking behaviour, and involvement in dangerous situations.

The assessment

This involves meeting with adolescent and parents using a comprehensive, systematic and sympathetic approach. The main aims are to ascertain:

- The number of substances used.
- Functional impairment, i.e. the effects of use on all areas of functioning such as social, family, cognitive, emotional, and academic.
- The presence of associated psychiatric and behavioural disorders and their temporal relationship to the substance use. This may require serial observations during periods of abstinence.

- The presence of family and environmental stresses including a past or present history of child abuse.
- The severity and extent of the problem, be it substance misuse or dependence.
- The highest level of functioning prior to illness.
- The perceived benefit of the substance and the concerns associated with discontinuation.
- Any adverse consequences on physical health, for example HIV and hepatitis infection.

In addition all adolescents presenting following an accident or trauma should be screened for substance use. The screening should include serum and urine samples. However a negative result does not exclude use as each drug has a different duration of detection after last use.

Management

The long term treatment goal of adolescents with substance use disorders is the maintenance of abstinence. In the short term where this is not possible harm reduction may be a more realistic goal. This may include the reduction of frequency and quantity of drug used and setting a goal to improve functioning such as interpersonal relationships and school performance. The most practical way to approach this is to consider their readiness to change. This a non-judgmental process of ascertaining motivation. There are five stages:

1. Precontemplation—denial of any problem or acknowledging its existence but not being willing to contemplate change.
2. Contemplation—acknowledging a problem but unwilling to tackle it.
3. Preparation—prepared to consider tackling the problem but not yet.
4. Action—willingness to tackle the problem.
5. Maintenance—working on maintaining gains.

In essence an assessment of needs should be matched with an appropriate package of care. Practical clinicians will try to:

- Identify the perceived benefits of the substance use.
- Identify the perceived disadvantages.
- Explore less harmful ways of achieving the benefits.
- Provide comprehensive, high quality care for all identified associated problems and comorbidity.
- Remove obstacles to progress.
- Reduce harm from substance abuse.
- Provide safe opportunities for withdrawal.
- Facilitate contact with self-help groups such as Alcoholics Anonymous for the adolescent and Al-Anon for the family.

Treatment setting

The treatment setting will depend on which is the least restrictive, safe and effective option, yet sensitive to the developmental needs of the child. Possibilities include inpatient care, residential treatment, day hospital, outpatient treatment, and community care. Other factors that need to be considered are the presence of medical or psychiatric conditions, the availability of services in the local area, the adolescent's and family's preference, and a history of failure in less restrictive treatment settings. Those with either a past history of withdrawal, or at risk of withdrawal, will most probably require an inpatient setting, as will children who are at risk to themselves, at risk to others, or who are acutely psychotic. Those with inadequate psychosocial support and a history of relapse following inpatient care may need to be considered for a residential placement, possibly following an inpatient detoxification. Adolescents with good family and social support who are at risk of relapse can be followed up as day patients. Those in need of less complicated combinations of treatment modalities may be best treated in an outpatient setting. Attendance at self-help or aftercare groups such as Alcoholics Anonymous are generally associated with improved outcome. There is no evidence currently to support the effectiveness of one treatment modality over another. Treatments available include individual or family approaches.

Treatment options

Motivational enhancement therapy

This is a transtheoretical approach to helping the adolescent achieve the motivation to give up substance use. It is based on the five stages of change outlined above. The focus of work is on the level of motivation rather than the substance misuse itself. The therapist explores patiently, sympathetically and non-judgementally the perceived benefits of the misuse. There is low investment in getting the adolescent to change but high investment in understanding the benefits. This non-coercive approach, skilfully applied, can ultimately have the paradoxical effect of encouraging expression of the perceived disadvantages and a wish to change. Once the action stage has been reached other therapies can be introduced.

Individual therapy

Cognitive behavioural therapy targets maladaptive thinking patterns, problem solving, anger control, relaxation training, and addresses relapse prevention. It allows the adolescent to learn strategies to deal with stressors and triggers that precede relapse. Interpersonal therapy may be useful for patients with comorbid depression and anxiety disorders. However, the golden rule with therapy is to focus on realistic ways to encourage coping with day to day life. Therapy which promotes insight, and therefore anxiety, should only be pursued after several years of stable living. Breaking this rule frequently leads to relapse.

Family interventions

Family interventions are an important part of the treatment package. Not only do family factors increase the risk of substance abuse, but also they can play an important part in determining outcome. Components of family work include education about the disorder, encouraging the family to support help-seeking behaviour in the adolescent, promoting limit setting, and improving communication and parental effectiveness. Therapy may also occur in groups of families with an emphasis on supporting and educating each other. Psychopathology existing in parents and child abuse may need identification and treatment in their own right.

Pharmacotherapy

Pharmacotherapy is commonly required for a number of reasons:

- For treating withdrawal symptoms in detoxification programmes.
- As substance substitution and craving reduction.
- For the treatment of drug induced psychosis and other psychiatric illnesses. Before medication is directed at any possible comorbid psychiatric disorder a period of abstinence from substances is usually recommended because these psychiatric disorders may well be secondary to the substance use. However, in practice there is a less than complete history, a less than perfect abstinence, and a less than perfect adherence to medication, with a steady working towards a more rational regimen.

Acamprosate and naltrexone may reduce crave and drinking related euphoria. Serotonin selective re-uptake inhibitors will help associated anxiety and depression. Monoamine oxidase inhibitors should be avoided in this population because of problems with interactions with alcoholic drinks containing tyramine and, more importantly in the young, the coattendant use of MDMA ("ecstasy").

Where possible medications should be chosen which will have a low potential for abuse overdose and which are given under close supervision.

Conclusion

There is a lot of opportunity for confusion and error in treating young people with substance abuse. Feelings of powerlessness and futility frequently hinder us from providing the basics and the necessary. The main goals are to keep therapeutic expectations and harm reduction low, and to allow time for maturity and changes in motivation to take place. Most of those who drink excessively during adolescence and young adulthood will moderate during their mid to late twenties. On average most heroin addicts will take 15 admissions for detoxification and subsequent relapse before they become abstinent in the longer term (usually in their late twenties or early thirties). The longer those with alcohol abuse or dependence live the more likely they will become abstinent provided they can be preserved from cognitive damage. Wasted years educationally, vocationally and interpersonally remain the most tangible legacy of substance use disorders together with the shame of antisocial and disinhibited behaviour and the scars of traumatic and traumatised relationships. Sympathetic and no-nonsense advice on how to rebuild a personal life and career realistically and incrementally is often much appreciated.

Further reading

American Academy of Child and Adolescent Psychiatry (AACAP) Official Action. Practice Parameters for the assessment and treatment of children and adolescents with substance use disorders. *Journal of the American Academy of Child and Adolescent Psychiatry* 1997;**36**:140S–56S.

Brizer D, Castaneda R. *Addiction and recovery for beginners*. London: Writers and Readers Publishing, 1996.

Fleisch B. *Approaches in the treatment of adolescents with emotional and substance abuse problems*. DHHS Publication ADM 91–1744. Washington, DC: US Government Printing Office, 1991.

8: Feeding and eating problems

Introduction

This chapter deals with the feeding problems of infancy and preschool children, the eating problems of childhood and the eating disorders which tend to arise in adolescence, and obesity.

Feeding problems of infancy and preschool children

Up to one third of mothers report problems feeding their infants and preschool children. Feeding problems of infancy and preschool children include problems of weaning, rumination, pica, and reluctance to eat specific foods (food faddiness) or any foods (food refusal).

Aetiology

Contributing causative factors in the child include:

- The presence of physical illness such as reflux vomiting, food intolerance, or colic
- Irritability or hyperactivity
- Trauma, especially associated with feeding.

Contributing causative factors in the family include:

- Inadequate milk production
- Marital disharmony
- Maternal ill health including disorders such as depression, anxiety, or eating disorder
- Attachment difficulties.

A vicious cycle may develop, where the parents respond to poor eating with increasing anxiety, leading to feeding becoming an aversive experience, with the child becoming more fraught and consuming less. Contributing causative factors in the environment include:

- Adverse living conditions such as overcrowding or poverty
- Poor social support and interfering relatives can hinder the feeding process and reduce parental confidence.

Specific problems and their treatments

Difficulties with weaning

Multiple factors may determine the age at which weaning occurs, including family and cultural norms, the need to return to work and breast feeding being used as a comforter. Some infants wean with ease, others are very resistant. In the latter case, treatment involves establishing a consistent routine with limits on the number of milk feeds, and a gradual reduction in the number of milk feeds per day, whilst increasing the number of other sources of fluid. Determination is sometimes required.

Rumination

Rumination, which can begin at any time during infancy or childhood, is the repeated regurgitation and re-chewing of food, followed by reswallowing or expulsion of the vomit, in the absence of a medical disorder. It is often associated with developmental delay. Urgent referral for behavioural treatment is required because of such complications as failure to thrive, haematemesis, dehydration, and dental caries.

Treatment of rumination often focuses on nutritional interventions, with satiating quantities of starchy food reducing after-meal rumination substantially. Manipulation of food quantities, increased stomach distention, increased caloric density, and increased oropharyngeal stimulation all have been shown to reduce after-meal rumination.

Pica

Pica is the frequent ingestion of non-nutritious substances, such as paper or paint, beginning between the ages of 12 and 24 months. It should not be confused with the transitional phase of mouthing in those less than 2 years of age. Pica is associated with developmental delay, autism, iron deficiency, Kleine–Levin syndrome, and parental neglect. Management involves treatment of the underlying cause and the consequences of the behaviour such as lead poisoning.

Food faddiness and food refusal

Food fads are so common in the second and third year of life that they can almost be considered to be developmentally normal. They consist of the toddler being very fussy about what to eat, and possibly accepting only a very few different foods. Generally toddlers grow out of this providing no fuss is made, but the behaviour may persist if too much attention is paid to it (see selective eating below).

Some young children show a reluctance to consume solid foods. This may occur as a result of delay in introducing solids or an aversive experience such as coercion. With sensible non-coercive management including a gradual introduction of solids, cutting the food into very small pieces and perhaps making a game of eating it, the problem usually resolves. Encouragement and rewards for success should be immediate and plentiful. Referral to a speech and language therapist may be required.

There is a group of young children who refuse food for no obvious reason and may simply have a rather poor appetite. In later childhood their parents will refer to them as always having been poor eaters. Some of these children manage to grow normally but others fail to thrive. On more detailed assessment this latter group may show quite severe emotional disturbance or emotional deprivation. Comprehensive assessment and treatment is indicated in these circumstances.

Management

A careful assessment of all feeding difficulties is indicated, especially when there is evidence of failure to thrive. The assessment should include:

- A dietary and developmental history
- An assessment of the child's nutritional status
- Exclusion of organic causes for failure to thrive
- Descriptions of a typical meal
- An exploration of the parent's expectations and attitudes towards food
- Observations of the mother–child relationship
- A diary of type and amount of food eaten over a few days
- Observations of a meal either on video or live. This is often very revealing of the underlying problem, not infrequently inappropriate parental management.

Many of these problems spontaneously resolve especially if handled without fuss or undue attention. Those that persist but are causing no harm, other than raising parental anxiety, are best allowed to resolve with time. If however there is evidence of impaired growth or health then parental counselling, a behavioural approach at meal times, plus attention to the underlying causes are all indicated.

Prognosis

Most of these children outgrow their feeding problem, although poor appetite and faddy eating can persist into later childhood and even adolescence.

Eating problems and disorders of childhood and adolescence

There are a number of conditions that tend to arise from the age of 5 upwards. Some are more likely to emerge prior to adolescence, for example food avoidance, emotional disorder, selective eating, functional dysphagia, and pervasive refusal syndrome, and are collectively described as eating problems of childhood. Others are more likely to occur in adolescence, for example anorexia nervosa and bulimia nervosa. However it is not unknown for the reverse to also occur. Anorexia nervosa and bulimia nervosa are collectively known as eating disorders. In this section we start with a description of the eating problems of childhood, followed by the eating disorders. Their aetiology and management is then discussed together. Finally we briefly discuss overeating and obesity.

Food avoidance emotional disorder (FAED)

FAED is a term used to describe children who have a primary emotional disorder in which food avoidance is a prominent feature. These children present with mood disturbance (mild depression, anxiety, obsessionality, or phobias), food avoidance, and significant weight loss. However they do not have the same preoccupation with, nor distortion of, weight and shape that is characteristic of anorexia nervosa. The weight loss can be as severe as in anorexia nervosa with all the accompanying physical complications. Many children with FAED have a physical illness and seem to develop food avoidance as a response to their ill health.

The incidence of FAED is unknown but is likely to be more common than that of anorexia nervosa (see below). It occurs more frequently in girls and generally has a good prognosis if treated correctly.

Selective eating

Selective eaters consume only a very narrow range of foods, commonly carbohydrate based, and are often very fussy about the brand of food, or where it was bought. Attempts to widen their range of foods are usually met with extreme distress and resistance. The children do not have a distorted body image, nor the preoccupation with weight or shape, characteristic of anorexia nervosa and bulimia nervosa. Growth and development in selective eaters does not appear to be affected by their eating habits. Selective eating may be a variant of normal eating behaviour, a failure to resolve the normal phase of food faddiness in toddlers, or an obsessional disorder. Parental requests for help occur at two ages. In childhood, selective eaters are usually referred because of parental concerns about the adequacy of nutrition, despite the fact that these children tend to thrive. In the early teens there is more concern about the impact the selective eating patterns have on social functioning. Although parents are able to manage the child's extreme fussiness by providing access to favoured foods at home, they are unable to do so once the child gets older and starts to take part in social events such as sleep-overs and school trips. Most selective eating problems tend to resolve during the teenage years as peer group influences become stronger and the need to conform in adolescence will often result in determined efforts to overcome their inability to eat normally.

Selective eating occurs far more commonly in boys than girls, and although the incidence is unknown, it is probably more common than anorexia nervosa.

Functional dysphagia

The characteristic feature of functional dysphagia is a fear of swallowing, vomiting, or choking, which makes the child anxious about, and resistant to eating normally, resulting in a marked avoidance of food. This avoidance tends to be foods of a certain type or texture. These children do not have the characteristic weight and shape concerns seen in patients with anorexia nervosa or bulimia nervosa. Usually there is an easily identifiable precipitant, such as having been force fed, witnessing someone choking whilst eating, having choked on a piece of food, or having had a traumatic gastrointestinal investigation.

The incidence is very low and it affects both sexes equally.

Pervasive refusal syndrome

Pervasive refusal syndrome is a potentially life-threatening condition manifested by a profound and pervasive refusal to eat, drink, walk, talk, or care for themselves in any way over a period of several months. These children usually present as underweight and often dehydrated, but it is unclear whether they have distorted cognitions regarding weight and shape, as they are unwilling to communicate. An additional and striking feature is their determined resistance to any form of help. The condition may represent an extreme form of post-traumatic stress disorder, possibly associated with learned helplessness. It is a rare condition, far more common in girls. Hospitalisation is almost always required and full recovery generally occurs, albeit often taking over a year.

Eating disorders

The eating disorders (anorexia nervosa and bulimia nervosa) are distinguished from the feeding and eating problems of childhood by a core disturbance in cognitions concerning body weight and shape. Specifically there is a morbid preoccupation with weight and shape accompanied by an unshakeable conviction of being overweight or fat and by poor self-esteem. These conditions arise most commonly in adolescence but can occur earlier, although never in preschool children.

Anorexia nervosa

Anorexia nervosa is characterised by determined attempts to lose weight or to avoid weight gain either by restricting food intake, self-induced vomiting, laxative abuse, excessive exercising, or more usually a combination of one or more of these. Although these patients tend to be high achievers, popular and conscientious, they usually have a poor self-image, feel ashamed of themselves, and have a sense of lacking control in their lives. There may be comorbid depression or obsessive compulsive disorder, and self-harm is not uncommon.

Boys present slightly differently from girls in that they tend to be more concerned about being "flabby" than fat, and want to become more muscular, rather than lose weight. They often equate being overweight with being unhealthy rather than unattractive. However, they are very similar to girls in that they avoid eating foods that they regard as fattening or unhealthy, and usually exercise excessively, with the end result being a significant weight loss. The physical complications of weight loss and the associated behaviours affect all the body systems. The most common problems include dehydration; cardiovascular abnormalities such as hypotension, bradycardia, and reduced peripheral circulation, with ensuing cold skin, acrocyanosis, delayed healing, dry skin and hair, and lanugo hair; parotid gland enlargement and dental erosion, both from repeated vomiting; loss of, or failure to develop, secondary sexual characteristics; carotenaemia; osteopenia and occasionally osteoporosis and impaired growth.

Demography In adolescence the prevalence of anorexia nervosa is about 0·1–0·2%, but much lower in children. It is likely that there has been an increase in the incidence in the last 40 years, and possible that it is continuing to increase. Between 90% and 95% of patients are female. The previously reported social class bias appears to be becoming less pronounced as time goes by and increasingly children and adolescents from ethnic minorities are being affected.

Prognosis and outcome The outcome for children and adolescents with anorexia nervosa is unsatisfactory with as many as 50% failing to make a complete recovery. Factors that appear to predict a good outcome include a good parental relationship and an ability on the child's part to express previously suppressed negative emotions.

Bulimia nervosa

Bulimia nervosa is very rare prepubertally but increasingly common during adolescence. As with adults it is characterised by episodes of overeating in which the sufferer experiences a loss of control. These episodes are usually followed by compensatory behaviours designed to avoid weight gain, for example, self-induced vomiting, laxative or diuretic abuse, excessive exercising, and periods of fasting or severe food restriction. The weight and shape concerns characteristic of anorexia nervosa are also core features of bulimia nervosa. Sufferers of bulimia nervosa often engage in self-harm, and have a very poor self-image.

Many bulimic women, who typically only present for treatment after many years of having the disorder, report that their bulimia started in early adolescence, suggesting that the disorder can remain "hidden" for a long time. Although bulimia nervosa has been reported in men there have been virtually no reports of it affecting prepubertal boys.

The physical complications are generally those associated with repeated vomiting, including parotid gland enlargement, dental erosion, oesophageal bleeding, and the development of polycystic ovaries.

Aetiology

Eating problems and disorders have a complex and multifactorial aetiology. Possible contributing factors include genetic, biological, psychological, personality, familial and sociocultural factors. Some, such as genetic and sociocultural influences, are necessary preconditions (predisposing factors) for anorexia nervosa and bulimia nervosa. Others act as precipitants, for example teasing about being overweight may precipitate anorexia nervosa or witnessing or experiencing an episode of choking may trigger functional dysphagia. Once the eating difficulty has emerged, the same or other factors may perpetuate it.

In summary a complex mix of factors contribute to the development of the eating difficulties and disorders. Furthermore some of these factors (for example, genetic, personality, biological) predispose to the illness (i.e. they are necessary preconditions for its emergence), others (for example, stressful events) precipitate the illness, and yet others (for example, the way in which the illness is managed) may perpetuate it. To complicate the situation further some factors (for example, family dysfunction) may both precipitate and perpetuate the illness.

Management

With regard to all the eating difficulties and disorders of childhood and adolescence, a comprehensive approach to treatment is essential. These problems have the potential to severely damage health, the patient often has a lack of insight into the seriousness of their illness, and there are often battles around control. It is vital therefore to create a therapeutic alliance with the primary carers providing them with information and education and helping them to take complete responsibility for the child's health until the child is well enough to take more of it for herself.

Assessment of the physical state is a priority with early rehydration and reversal of any electrolyte imbalance. Refeeding and weight restoration are also early goals. The restoration of normal eating patterns is an intermediate aim, along with addressing the underlying intra- and interpersonal problems that may have contributed to and helped to maintain the illness.

The sine-qua-non of the treatment programme is parental counselling, often in association with family therapy. Individual approaches to treatment should include attention to motivational enhancement as well as problem focussed or cognitive behavioural techniques. Resistance to treatment is such that without working on improving motivation other approaches will have limited success. Psychodynamic methods are best reserved for deeply entrenched problems that remain unalleviated by other approaches.

There is a limited role only for psychotropic medication in this population. Antidepressants such as the SSRIs (selective serotonin reuptake inhibitors) can be helpful if there is clinical evidence of depression, and also in bulimia nervosa. Anxiolytics may have some limited value when anxiety levels are high. However they should be used sparingly. Vitamins, calcium and other essential nutrients may be used to supplement a poor diet. Laxatives should not be used as a first line treatment for constipation, which is best managed by dietary means. Oestrogens should not be used to initiate menstruation, although they may have a part to play if osteporosis has developed.

The establishment of normal eating patterns is not a high priority but a healthy dietary intake is essential. This is best achieved in consultation with the child, parents and if necessary a dietitian. Whatever techniques are used they must be applied consistently between the carers and consistently over time. This is most likely to occur if the carers are in agreement with each other about how to proceed and as comfortable as possible with the techniques chosen.

Transabdominal pelvic ultrasound is the best means of determining whether the weight gain is sufficient in girls, as target weights are often set far too low, with the danger of persisting amenorrhoea and its long term complications. For boys population norms are the only standard available. In general, children will need to achieve a body mass index (BMI) of 19·5 or more to ensure they are within a healthy range.

Hospitalisation is indicated when there is dehydration that has not been reversed within 24 hours, electrolyte imbalance, peripheral circulatory collapse, a BMI below 14, severe depression, suicidal behaviour, or failed outpatient treatment.

Obesity

Obesity is defined as an excess of body fat and occurs when the BMI exceeds the 90th centile. Prevalence rates vary between countries, with rates as high as 28% reported in 6–11 year olds in the USA. Girls and those from lower socioeconomic classes are more at risk. Most obese children are likely to be genetically predisposed to gain weight more readily and for some environmental factors such as family patterns of overeating or the tendency to use food as a comfort are likely to aggravate the problem. Most obese children are concerned about their obesity but do not manifest their concern in the same way as those with anorexia nervosa or bulimia nervosa. They certainly are not tormented to the same degree and make minimal effort to lose weight. They do however have in common with those with eating disorders, denial, a strong tendency to very poor self-esteem, and resistance to treatment.

Management

As with any of the eating difficulties and disorders treatment needs to be comprehensive. Indeed there is a surprising degree of overlap, whether attempts are being made to increase or decrease food intake. The parents should be central to the treatment programme whilst individual approaches should include a strong focus on enhancing motivation as well as dealing with such issues as poor self-esteem. Education about healthy eating and energy expenditure may have a place but, in the absence of enhancing motivation, will have no effect. Low calorie diets and increased exercise are obviously necessary but insufficient on their own. Older children may benefit from groups such as "WeightWatchers". Surgery should be reserved for those with metabolic diseases or life-threatening complications.

Prognosis

Obesity is remarkably intractable despite many treatments appearing to help in the short term. However weight gain is all too common after treatment stops. Around 40% of obese children remain obese in adulthood. Long term risks include cardiovascular disease, hypertension, diabetes, emphysema, digestive diseases, and increased operative risk. The prognosis is likely to be improved by the adoption of a comprehensive approach to treatment with a focus on motivation and self-esteem, and treatments being curtailed only very gradually over a period of several months, and only after there is good evidence of sustained weight loss.

Further reading

Bryant-Waugh R, Lask B. *Eating disorders—a parents' guide*. London: Penguin, 1999.
Flodmark C-E. Childhood obesity. *Clinical Child Psychology and Psychiatry* 1997;2:283–95.
Hodes M. Feeding disorders. *Prescribers' Journal* 1995;35:192–8.
Lask B, Bryant-Waugh R, eds. *Anorexia nervosa and related eating disorders in childhood and adolescence*. Hove, UK: Psychology Press, 2000.

9: Habits, mannerisms, tics, obsessions and compulsions

Introduction

Habits and mannerisms, tics, obsessions and compulsions are common phenomena in childhood and sometimes occur in association with each other.

Habits and mannerisms

These include head-banging, hair-pulling, rocking, thumb-sucking, and nail-biting. It is likely that there is a genetic component to such behaviours, which are commonly aggravated by stress. They are probably more common in those with a learning disability (see chapter 15). In general they are self-limiting, especially if no fuss is made. They are relatively harmless, although those with head-banging require careful observation and safety precautions. The cosmetic consequences of hair-pulling (trichotillomania) can be problematic and occasionally the hair is swallowed producing hairballs (trichobezoar) which can cause intestinal obstruction.

Treatment is generally organised around behavioural techniques (see chapter 24) but parental counselling is always indicated. Occasionally medication for anxiety (see chapter 25) may be necessary.

Tics

Tics are paroxysmal, sudden, rapid, repetitive, involuntary, non-rhythmic movements, gestures or utterances. There may or may not be conscious awareness and, with effort, can sometimes be suppressed from seconds to hours. Tics vary in severity and may be subdivided into simple and complex.

Simple tics are abrupt movements involving only one muscle group such as eye blinking, head jerks, or shoulder shrugs. Simple vocal tics result from the passage of air through vocal chords, nasal passages, and pharynx, and include grunting, sniffing, and throat clearing.

Complex tics involve a number of muscle groups and result in more purposeful behaviours such as facial expressions or gestures of the arms or head. These movements can involve obscene gestures (copropraxia) or self-injury, for example hitting or biting. Complex vocal tics include vocalisations such as repetition of heard phrases (echolalia), repetition of one's own words or sounds (palilalia), or utterances of obscenities (coprolalia).

Tourette's syndrome is characterised by a combination of complex motor and vocal tics, and may also involve coprolalia, copropraxia, attention deficit, impulsivity, and obsessive compulsive features.

Epidemiology

Mild tics affect up to 10% of children, complex tics are considerably less common, and Tourette's syndrome occurs in about 1 in 2000. Tics occur in all races and social classes and are more common in boys by a ratio of 4 to 1 in Tourette's Syndrome. Onset is usually in early childhood although Tourette's syndrome only becomes evident between about 7 and 10 years.

Aetiology

Tics are probably genetically determined with external stress factors precipitating and aggravating them. The concordance figures for Tourette's syndrome among monozygotic twins is greater than 50% and dizygotic twins only 10%. Other factors may contribute to the development of these conditions but currently have not been clearly delineated.

Clinical features

Typically tics initially affect one muscle group, such as the face or neck. They may then resolve completely, persist, or progress to affect other muscle groups, either singly or in combination, and may be motor, vocal or both. The diagnosis of Tourette's syndrome is often made on the basis of severity but usually includes complex motor and vocal tics. Echolalia, coprolalia and copropraxia are not core features and occur in about half of the children with Tourette's syndrome at some point during their illness.

Though initially in Tourette's syndrome there is a fluctuating course, with addition or replacement of symptoms, eventually they may become persistent, resulting in significant distress and disability.

By the age of 10 most children are aware of the premonitory urge that precedes the tics. Awareness may contribute to the ability to suppress the tic for a longer period of time. Exacerbating factors include stress and drugs such as stimulants. Tics can be curbed by sleep, relaxation, alcohol, and intense concentration.

Comorbidity

Comorbid conditions include obsessive compulsive symptoms (see below), attention deficit, hyperactivity, anxiety, behaviour difficulties, sleep disturbance, depression, and self-injurious behaviour.

Differential diagnosis

This includes obsessive compulsive disorder, myoclonic epilepsy, Sydenham's chorea, Wilson's disease, and Huntingdon's chorea.

Treatment

Children with transient tic disorders, unless severe, require only reassurance, with a statement that tics are common and likely to disappear, especially if ignored. For the more severe tic disorders the mainstays of treatment includes parental counselling (see chapter 22), cognitive behavioural therapy (see chapter 24), and various medications (see chapter 25). Coexisting psychiatric problems should receive the appropriate treatment including cognitive behavioural therapy for the associated anxiety and to improve social functioning.

It is important to advise parents that the condition usually improves over time, and this is more likely if the tics can be ignored. The capacity to suppress the tics is often taken as evidence of a voluntary behaviour, therefore it is also important to emphasise their involuntary nature. Similar advice should be given to teachers, cautioniong against any negative attitudes. Information can be given to the child's peers to improve their understanding of the condition. It is best presented within the school setting as part of a broader health education perspective.

Support groups for parents and children have proved both popular and helpful.

Pharmacological treatments should be used if there is significant impairment, stigmatisation, or strong intolerance. Clonidine is usually the first line medication, particularly when attention deficit hyperactivity disorder is also present. Its advantage is its absence of long term side effects. However it has a suboptimal efficacy with a significant proportion of patients reporting little or no improvement. Clomipramine, sertraline and fluoxetine are used when obsessive compulsive behaviour is prominent or when the tic treatment is inadequate. Haloperidol is amongst the most effective agents but does have powerful side effects including weight gain, acute dystonia, cognitive dulling, tremor, akathesia, and later tardive dyskinesia. Pimozide is no longer recommended because of its potential for affecting cardiac conduction. Other neuroleptics of value include risperidone and sulpiride.

Tics and Tourette's syndrome wax and wane, therefore treatment should not be adjusted quickly or frequently. Individual tics will have a phasic life of roughly 6–12 weeks. It is best not to adjust medication following worsening of symptoms unless the exacerbation has persisted for a few weeks or the tics are causing impairment in functioning. The efficacy of medication may reduce with time and under such circumstances it is helpful to alternate the drugs used. In more severe cases combination medication may help.

The anticipation of relapse and remission is an important component if coping with chronicity.

Course and prognosis

The prognosis for simple tics is good, for complex tics moderate, and rather poorer for Tourette's syndrome. There is an improvement with age, with the first 10 years of Tourette's being the worst. By late adolescence or early adulthood, tics remit almost completely in about one third of cases, and an additional one third will show significant reduction in both frequency and severity, with the remaining third continuing to be symptomatic in adulthood. The comorbid features such as attention deficit, impulsivity, and obsessive compulsive features often persist into adult life.

Obsessive compulsive disorder in children and adolescents

Definitions

Obsessions are recurrent, persistent, intrusive thoughts, images or impulses, frequently acknowledged as senseless, and resulting in distress to the individual. Affected children will attempt to ignore, suppress or neutralise obsessive thoughts and associated feelings by "performing compulsions".

Compulsions are repetitive, purposeful behaviours, performed in response to an obsession, often in a stereotypical fashion. These compulsions lead to great distress for all involved.

Obsessive compulsive disorder is characterised by recurrent obsessions and/or compulsions that cause marked distress and/or interference.

Epidemiology

Obsessions and compulsions occur commonly as normal aspects of development (for example avoiding cracks in pavements), and are best considered as superstitions or habits. They should only be considered as pathological when they cause distress. Obsessive compulsive disorder affects between 0·5% and 1% of the younger population but the disorder frequently goes unrecognised, as children tend to be secretive about their difficulties. It is unclear at what age obsessions might commence, but they are rarely evident in prepubertal children. The gender ratio is equal.

Aetiology

Genetic factors are likely to be the main contributor with evidence of strong family histories in those affected and from twin studies. Brain imaging commonly demonstrates abnormalities of the basal ganglia, suggesting a neurobiological substrate. There is also increasing evidence for the possibility of a recent streptococcal infection in a subgroup who have a sudden onset with no previous history. Stress aggravates preexisting symptoms.

Clinical symptoms

Whilst isolated obsessions or compulsions do occur, more commonly they present in combination. Common obsessional themes include contamination, aggression, sex, and religion, and the urge to carry out certain activities in a repetitive, specific and ritualised manner. Common compulsions include repetition, washing, checking, touching, counting, and ordering. There is invariably considerable associated anxiety, and anger or even aggression when thwarted. Parents often become caught up in complex rituals to avoid upsetting their child.

Comorbidity

Comorbid conditions include: habits, trichotillomania, tics, and Tourette's syndrome (see above), anxiety disorders (see chapter 3), depressive disorders (see chapter 6), anorexia nervosa (see chapter 8), disruptive disorder (see chapter 5), autistic spectrum disorder (see chapter 16), and learning difficulties.

Differential diagnosis

This includes autistic spectrum disorder (see chapter 16) and anorexia nervosa and other eating disorders (see chapter 8).

Treatment

This consists of a comprehensive approach including parental counselling (see chapter 22), cognitive behavioural therapy (see chapter 24), and medication (see chapter 25). Parents should be encouraged to reduce their preoccupation with the symptoms per se and focus on the social needs of the child. If they can steadily reduce their tendency to accommodate to the compulsions in a firm but gentle and non-punitive manner, symptoms may well reduce and eventually resolve.

Cognitive behavioural therapy is considered by some to be the treatment of choice in adults, and it is likely to be of considerable value in the younger population. The goal of treatment is to have the child in control of the disorder rather than the disorder in control of the child. Full details are provided in chapter 24.

Medication also has considerable value in up to two thirds of patients, although it may take up to 12 weeks to have an effect. Antidepressants with a principle action at serotonergic synapses (for example clomipramine), and the SSRIs (for example sertraline, fluoxetine, and fluvoxamine) are more effective in reducing obsessional symptoms than non-serotonergic antidepressants. Complex medication combinations should be avoided until there has been a complete trial of single medication, cognitive behavioural therapy, and parental counselling. Combinations might include clomipramine with either clonazepam (for patients with high levels of anxiety) or haloperidol/risperidone (particularly for those with tics or thought disorder symptoms), or SSRIs with buspirone, fenfluramine, trazadone, a benzodiazepine, haloperidol, or risperidone.

Prognosis

The outcome is rather poor. Among adults with obsessive compulsive disorder one third to one half have developed the disorder during childhood. About half improve over 2–7 years, but many relapse when medication is withdrawn. However, cognitive behavioural therapy may reduce relapse on discontinuation of medication. Specialist clinics for obsessive compulsive disorder are reporting increasingly optimistic findings, especially in those of later onset with less comorbidity and family pathology.

Further reading

Leckman JF, Cohen D. Tic disorders. In: Rutter M, Taylor E, Hersov L, eds. *Child and adolescent psychiatry. Modern approaches*, 3rd edn. Oxford: Blackwell Science, 1994:455–65.

Mash J, Leonard H. Obsessive-compulsive disorder in children and adolescents. A review of the past 10 years. *Journal of the American Academy of Child and Adolescent Psychiatry* 1996;**34**:1266–71.

McGuire P. The brain in obsessive-compulsive disorder. *Journal of Neurology, Neurosurgery and Psychiatry* 1995;**59**:457–9.

10: Sleep problems

Introduction

Sleep problems are common and can be exhausting and demoralising for all concerned. It is important to distinguish between physiologically normal sleep and disturbed sleep. It is usually possible to make a diagnosis on the basis of careful history-taking alone, but sometimes physical examination and investigations are required. Parental support is essential and platitudes such as "just a phase" or "he will grow out of it" should be avoided.

Normal sleep in childhood

A newborn may sleep from 14 hours to 20 hours in 4–6 hour stretches over the course of 24 hours. At 3 months 70% will sleep through the night, at 6 months 85%, and at 1 year 90% will be sleeping continuously through the night. By 18 months this will be on average reduced to 14 hours, at 30 months 12 hours, and 5 years 9–11 hours.

Sleep can be divided into REM (rapid eye movement sleep), during which dreaming and muscle relaxation occur, and NREM which can be further subdivided into four stages, 1, 2, 3, and 4. Sleep begins with NREM stages 1–4 progressing to REM and then back to NREM at 50-minute cycles in early childhood and 90-minute cycles in later childhood and adult life. These cycles are repeated 4–6 times during the night with increasing proportions of REM sleep towards the end of the night.

Sleep problems

In the first year of life night waking is so common that it can be considered as normal. There will however be additional factors that contribute, including colic, illness, noise, hunger, thirst, or discomfort from a soiled nappy or being too hot or cold. Calm and brief attention to such factors is usually sufficient. Too much stimulus is likely to aggravate sleep disturbance and taking the baby in to the parental bed is best avoided as this can be difficult to reverse. Consistency between parents and over time is important. Persistent sleep disturbance may require some low key assessment. It is important to exclude ill health and to ensure adequate nutrition. Parental stress or distress may be contributing, and a vicious cycle is easily generated when sleep deprivation occurs. Parental sharing of attention to night time problems makes an important difference.

In older children much the same rules apply. If attention is required this should always be as low key as possible and the older the child, the easier it is to apply rules. Some parents may wish to "sit out" the crying and those who do not should use increasing time gaps between crying and responding to the child. Long naps during the day and too much excitement at bedtime should be avoided. A regular bedtime routine such as set times for bathing, toileting, tucking in and bedtime story are all helpful adjuncts. When sleep disturbance is intractable more detailed support for the parents may be required (see chapter 22) and mild sedation such as chloral or other sedation (see chapter 25) may be used as a temporary measure.

When anxiety about being left alone is causing difficulties a graded approach to separation can be used (see chapter 24). For example initially a parent helps the child to settle and then stays beside the bed until sleep intervenes. Once this pattern has been established over several nights, the parent may then settle the child and stay in the room, but not by the bedside, until the child is asleep. After a few more nights the parent settles the child, and then stays outside the room, calmly reassuring the child but not re-entering the room. This graded approach can be adapted as necessary to fit different circumstances.

Nightmares

Nightmares occur during REM sleep, and the child awakes anxious, oriented, and with vivid recall of the dream. They affect almost all children occasionally and will recur intermittently through childhood and sometimes into adult life. They should not be considered abnormal and no treatment is required unless they are occurring very frequently (for example more than once a week). In such cases it is a good idea to avoid frightening stimuli such as certain stories or television programmes. A narrative approach can be tried in which the child is helped, by talking or drawing, to change the content of the dreams to include a triumphant ending.

Night terrors

Night terrors are recurrent episodes of abrupt partial awakening from sleep, with screaming and marked autonomic arousal, including flushing, tachycardia, tachypnoea, sweating, dilated pupils, and piloerection. The child is uncontactable and inconsolable during the episode and has no recall of it in the morning. The night terrors may be associated with sleepwalking (see below). The episodes occur typically during the first 3 hours of sleep (in deep NREM) usually at the same time of night, unlike nightmares which tend to occur in the latter part of the night during REM sleep. There is usually a "prodromal" period of about 15 minutes during which the signs of autonomic arousal may be observed. The episodes tend to last between 10 and 20 minutes, and rarely occur more than once a night. Night terrors commonly start around the age of 5–6, affect about 3% of children, and usually resolve by adolescence, with only 5% of those affected still having terrors in adult life. There is sometimes a family history of similar episodes, but there is no evidence of associated psychopathology, stressors, or family dysfunction.

The differential diagnosis incudes nightmares (see above) and epilepsy. However a careful history and description of the episodes is almost always sufficient to make the diagnosis. In nightmares, in addition to occurring later on in the night, the child is easier to wake, talk to, and console. Convulsions do not normally occur during the first 3 hours of sleep, the movements are more likely to be tonic clonic in nature, and intense vocalisation is rare. An EEG should be performed when doubt exists.

Treatment

Too often parents are told "not to worry", "they will disappear with time", and other such platitudes. Whilst usually true the terrors still need treatment because they are not only a source of much concern but also tend to interfere with the sleep of everyone within hearing distance. The mainstay of treatment is known as "the waking treatment". The parents are asked to keep a diary for a few nights to ascertain the pattern of episodes, noting the time of onset of the autonomic arousal and the time of the actual terror. Subsequently they should wake the child at the point autonomic arousal starts, or if they have not been able to ascertain this, then 10–15 minutes before the night terror usually occurs. If there is no consistent pattern and no evidence of autonomic arousal, then the child should be woken 10–15 minutes before the earliest recorded night terror. The child should be fully woken and kept awake for at least 5 minutes. This process is continued for between 5 and 7 days. If terrors do not occur or stop during this process the child should still be woken for the duration of the treatment period at the usual onset time.

Medication, such as the benzodiazepines (for example clonazepam which is usually first line administered for 3 months at adequate doses and then weaned with 70% effectiveness) should be reserved for those in whom the waking treatment fails. Carbamazepine may be used as an alternative. There is no evidence that psychotherapies are beneficial, although parental support is of course mandatory.

Sleep-walking (somnambulism)

Sleep-walking has much in common with night terrors (see above). Indeed it is probably only the behavioural manifestations that differ, and in some, both sleep-walking and night terrors occur. Up to a third of all children have had one episode of sleep-walking, though it occurs regularly in only 2·5%. Peak incidence is between 5 and 7 years, the rate declining after 9 years of age. Like night terrors the child appears unaware, fails to respond to questioning, and is difficult to wake with amnesia of the event in the morning. The parents should be advised to guide the child back to bed and to use safety precautions around the bed such as a bottom bunk, no heater, and bolting doors and windows leading to the outside. Although the waking treatment has not been evaluated it should certainly be tried using the same techniques as with night terrors. Medication is best reserved for intractable or extreme cases. The prognosis is good with remittance in the majority.

Hypersomnias

Hypersomnias describe those situations in which the child sleeps excessively during the day interfering with usual daytime activities. There are a number of conditions in which it occurs. These include the relatively common general tendency to daytime somnolence and the rarer causes of narcolepsy, Kleine–Levin syndrome, sleep apnoea, severe depression, substance abuse, endocrine and metabolic disorders, non-convulsive status epilepticus, and menstrual associated hypersomnia.

Daytime somnolence, the tendency to sleep during the day, affects 5% of the population with an onset in adolescence occurring particularly in boys. There are a number of contributory factors including: reduced nocturnal sleep resulting from social engagements and the additive effects of chronic sleep loss.

Narcolepsy involves the irresistible urge to sleep, including during the daytime, and sometimes associated with cataplexy (sudden loss of muscle tone) and hallucinations. The daytime sleep occurs several times a day lasting from 5 to 30 minutes followed by complete alertness. In addition, there may be "microsleeps" lasting a few seconds, during which the eyes are open but not responding and speech is unintelligible. Sometimes sleep paralysis occurs, at either the onset or termination of sleep, with the child being awake but immobile. Hallucinations may occur on falling asleep (hypnogogic) or on waking (hypnopompic) in 25% of those with narcolepsy. It should be noted that such hallucinations also occur occasionally in the normal population. They are generally frightening in nature. Narcolepsy seriously intrudes on normal living with schooling performance deteriorating sometimes dramatically and socialising suffering.

Narcolepsy is rarely diagnosed before 10 years of age, with onset most commonly in late adolescence. The incidence is around 0·02–0·09% of the population. It is more frequent where there is a family history, which is found in 40%. Associated epilepsy has been found in 10% of those with narcolepsy.

The diagnosis is made on the basis of the history and supportive evidence can be obtained from an EEG in which sleep onset REM or reduction in time in onset of the first REM sleep period can be seen.

Differential diagnosis includes sleep apnoea, hypothyroidism, hypoglycaemia, anaemia, uraemia, adrenal insufficiency, epilepsy, sleep deprivation and other psychiatric disorders such as depression and conversion disorders.

Treatment in the first instance should include regular 20-minute napping at lunchtime and after school. Diet manipulation using a low carbohydrate diet is used for older children. Stresses should be identified and teachers advised to make appropriate allowances. Medications (see chapter 25) worth trying include stimulants such as methylphenidate for the sleepiness and tricyclics such as clomipramine for the cataplexy.

The prognosis is poor with the problem being life long with high levels of comorbidity.

Kleine–Levin syndrome

Kleine–Levin syndrome is a rare disorder of unknown aetiology in which daytime somnolence is associated with hyperphagia (increased eating) and behavioural disturbance. It occurs particularly in boys towards the end of adolescence (median 16 years). The condition occurs suddenly often following an upper respiratory tract infection or a flu-like illness with fever, vomiting, photophobia and irritability, and outbreaks last only a few weeks with marked periodicity, i.e. intermittent hypersomnolence. The disorder has also been reported following head injury and dental anaesthesia. Behavioural disturbances can be diverse and include disorientation, disorder of mood, hyperactivity, sexual disinhibition, aggression, autistic features, and hallucinations. The EEG during an episode may show diffuse paroxysmal slowing.

Treatment is far from universally effective but it is worth trying lithium, carbamazepine, tricyclic antidepressants, or stimulants (see chapter 25).

Spontaneous remission usually occurs within several years.

Sleep apnoea

Sleep apnoea is arrest of breathing in sleep (i.e. absence of two respiratory cycles) and frequent waking. Sleep apnoea can be classified as having an obstructive, central or mixed aetiology. Obstructive sleep apnoea may be due to enlarged tonsils, adenoids, facial dysmorphism, neuromuscular disorder, or obesity. Snoring is a common accompaniment of obstructive sleep apnoea. Central sleep apnoea involves the absence of airflow at the mouth and movement of the chest wall. In a mixed picture the apnoea starts as central progressing to obstructive.

Subsequent behavioural problems due to sleep deprivation such as anxiety, depression and impaired school performance may all complicate the picture.

Investigations should include soft tissue x-rays of the lateral neck, chest x-ray, ECG, and arterial blood gas analysis. The diagnosis can be made by using a polysomnogram recording respiratory movement, expired carbon dioxide and pulse oximetry during sleep, together with a thorough ENT examination. Where there is doubt about the aetiology referral to a sleep specialist should be made.

Treatment includes directing attention to any anatomical cause for obstruction. This may involve weight reduction or removal of the tonsils and adenoids.

Nasal continuous posture airways pressure (CPAP) may be necessary at night.

Conclusions

Sleep disturbance in childhood is very common and may vary in aetiology from normal behaviour through to the potentially life threatening. Accurate diagnosis is an essential prerequisite to the advice and treatment offered. Platitudes should be avoided. Parental support is essential because they are so often themselves exhausted. Behavioural approaches and medication are the other mainstays of treatment.

Further reading

Lask B. Night terrors—a novel and non-toxic treatment. *British Medical Journal* 1988;**297**:592.

Pike M, Stores G. Kleine–Levin syndrome: a cause of diagnostic confusion. *Archives of Disease in Childhood* 1994;**71**:355–7.

Shaeffer C. *Clinical handbook of sleep disorders*. New York: Jason Aronson, 1995.

11: Enuresis and encopresis

Enuresis

Definition and classification

Enuresis is the involuntary emptying of the bladder subsequent to the expected age of usual bladder control. It can be divided into nocturnal, diurnal, or a combination of the two, and primary (a failure to establish continence) or secondary (a loss of continence following at least six months of dry nights).

Epidemiology

The development of control may be delayed, in particular where there is a strong family history. The majority of children are dry by night at the age of three years, 90% are dry at five years, 95% at 10 years, and 99% at 15. Nocturnal enuresis is more frequent than diurnal enuresis. Enuresis is twice as common in boys as in girls and there is a slightly increased rate in those from lower socioeconomic groups. Diurnal enuresis is more common in girls and in children with psychiatric disturbance. Enuresis over 10 years of age is almost always associated with significant psychosocial disruption and/or an organic substrate.

Aetiology

A number of factors may contribute, including:

- Family history of bed wetting—this occurs in approximately 70%
- General developmental delay
- Small bladder capacity
- Stressful life events (for example, separation, birth of younger sibling, trauma, hospitalisation)

- Social disadvantage (for example, family disorganisation or neglect and subsequent lack of appropriate training)
- Delay in initiation of toilet training.

Associated conditions

A number of comorbid disorders may be noted:

- Urinary tract infection (UTI) occurs in about 5%.
- Abnormalities of urinary tract including incomplete bladder voiding and a hypertrophic bladder wall are sometimes found in diurnal enuresis.
- Constipation, with resultant pressure on the bladder, may result in detrusor instability and enuresis.
- Associated psychiatric disorders; these present only in a minority, but are between two and six times more common than in non-enuretics. They occur particularly in girls, diurnal and secondary enuresis.

Management

Associated organic conditions should be excluded. Uncomplicated cases may respond to a simple programme of omitting drinks four hours before bed time, ensuring bladder emptying at bed time, and waking the child to repeat bladder emptying at the parent's bed time. It is important to ensure that the parents do not have a punitive attitude. Should this approach not work, a combination of parental counselling (see chapter 22), and behaviour therapy (see chapter 24) is usually sufficient.

Reward schemes are commonly used.

For example, star charts are a good way of emphasising a child's achievements as well as documenting progress. At least in the early phase, stars should be easily earned.

Enuresis alarms, commonly known as the "bell and pad", are appropriate for children over 6 years. A pad is placed under the sheet, which rings as soon as it becomes damp. The child should wake in consequence and is encouraged to complete urinating in the toilet. This approach requires a strong degree of parental motivation and organisation. These alarms are successful in approximately 80–90% of children after a few weeks, but have a relapse rate of up to 40%. In some cases the child sleeps through the alarm.

Diurnal wetting can be improved using gradually increasing intervals between voiding of urine. For example, on day 1 the child is encouraged to pass urine hourly, on day 2 every 1·5 hours, on day 3 every 2 hours, etc., until 3–4 hour intervals have been reached. Again organisation and motivation are required.

Medications

Medications may have considerable value, especially if used in combination with behavioural approaches and parental counselling. Tricyclics such as imipramine can be prescribed for a maximum 4–6 weeks. They are particularly useful for short periods, for example staying the night with a friend, or going on a trip, when it is important for the child to be dry. Relapse after ceasing medications is common. Desmopressin, an antidiuretic with few side effects, is an easy to use alternative. It is administered as a nasal spray, starting with 10 micrograms and gradually increasing the dose to 40 micrograms according to response. Treatment with desmopressin is recommended in older children who have not responded to behavioural interventions and may also be of particular use in known responders for short-term circumstances such as sleeping away from home.

Prognosis

The majority of children with enuresis are dry before or during adolescence. A very small minority will continue to wet into adulthood. Such children usually have severe associated problems.

Encopresis

Definition

Encopresis is the passage of faeces into inappropriate places, for example clothing or the bed. There are three main types:

- Primary encopresis in which bowel control has never been achieved.
- Secondary encopresis which occurs after bowel control has been achieved.
- Constipation with overflow in which the soiling is due to faecal impaction and leakage of fluid faeces.

Developmental considerations

In infancy, rectal emptying is an automatic response to the gastrocolic reflexes, resulting in stool production after a feed. Most children are physiologically able to gain bowel control between 18 and 24 months of age. Together with a desire by the child and positive reinforcement by the parents, this sets the stage for bowel control.

Epidemiology

Encopresis is more common in boys (ratio 3 or 4 : 1) and affects approximately 1% of school age children. Children from lower socioeconomic groups are more often affected and psychiatric disturbance is common.

Aetiology

Primary encopresis is generally associated with neglect, disadvantage, or developmental delay.

Secondary encopresis usually occurs after a stressor such as the birth of a sibling or separation. Occasionally it is associated with oppositional behaviour. There may be concomitant smearing of faeces and deliberate depositing away from the toilet. In such cases there are usually multiple associated problems for both the child and the family. Other forms of regressive behaviour such as clinging may occur. Comorbid disorders may include enuresis (see above), attention deficit hyperactivity disorder (see chapter 5), depression (see chapter 6), disruptive behaviour (see chapter 5), and speech delay (occurs in approximately 24%).

Retention with overflow occurs in approximately two thirds of encopretics where there is associated chronic constipation, faecal impaction, and overflow incontinence (retentive encopresis). Both physical and psychological factors contribute to the aetiology.

Physical factors include hardening of the stools from deficiency of fibre and fluids or from delay in opening the bowels. When the child defecates the passage of the hard, large stool may tear the anal mucosa and even ultimately create a fissure. The child may then delay further defecation with consequent anal spasm. The further holding onto the stools results in hardening and expansion of the stool with more pain on defecation, reconfirming the belief that defecation is painful. Furthermore, tension may impair relaxation of the voluntary muscle.

In studies of chronically constipated children, up to 75% have a history of painful defecation, and over half have blood in the stools. As many as 70% have associated faecal incontinence, with half becoming continuous soilers.

Toilet phobia

Secondary encopresis and retention with overflow may both be associated with a toilet phobia. The child avoids sitting on the toilet for fear of, for example, falling in or of a monster. Subsequently there is either constipation with overflow or soiling in the child's bed or clothing.

Management

Organic conditions such as Hirshspung's disease should be excluded and the possibility of child sexual abuse should always be considered. Physical examination for an anal fissure in constipated children is important, but rectal examination, which may be traumatic, is best avoided. Severe constipation can usually be diagnosed by abdominal examination.

The mainstays of treatment are a combination of parental counselling (see chapter 22), behaviour therapy (see chapter 24), and medication for those who are constipated. The nature of the disorder should be explained to the child and parents, and anatomical illustrations used to help understanding. Reassurance should be offered both to the child and parents—although the problem may have been longstanding, it is not necessarily intractable.

Common misunderstandings include:

- The fact that it takes 3 days for the bowel to refill. In this time period it may be thought that the child is again constipated when in fact the bowel is empty.
- Fluid faeces due to impaction and overflow may be thought to be due to diarrhoea.
- It may take a few months for retraining and retoning of the bowel and during this time the stool needs to be kept soft.

It is important to engage the cooperation of both parent and child in order to carry out a successful behavioural programme, as it requires persistence and consistency on all parts. Sometimes parental anger and frustration may impede the success of a treatment programme.

Another helpful approach is that known as "externalisation". The parents are encouraged to objectify and personify the problem. In encopresis the problem has been labelled as "sneaky poo", a fantasised object which "sneakily causes a poo to appear". The parents and child are then encouraged to join forces to overcome "sneaky poo". The humour inherent to such an approach neutralises or reduces some of the associated negative feelings.

Medication

Any constipation needs to be treated using high fibre diet and laxatives such as bulk or stool softeners, for example sorbitol, lactulose and methyl cellulose, and/or a stimulating agent such as senna. In resistant cases or where hard stools are palpable on abdominal examination, docusate (a stimulant and softening agent) should be used. Where necessary, suppositories or even enemas can be considered, but care must be taken to administer them in a sensitive way.

Subsequent routine bowel opening needs to be established with senna, and toileting routines. When feasible, laxatives are replaced by a high fibre diet. Withdrawal of any medication should be gradual and usually over several weeks. Abrupt or precipitate withdrawal almost invariably leads to relapse.

Behaviour modification (see also chapter 24)

It is important to emphasise to the parents that punitive approaches are counterproductive. In those who have never been toilet trained this should be initiated using a behaviour modification programme by the parents. The child is encouraged to spend 10 minutes on the toilet after meals without any pressure to produce stools, and should be rewarded subsequently. Further positive reinforcement for passing a stool appropriately and not soiling clothing is given. Star charts with rewards can be used as incentives, ensuring that the targets are achievable. Where continence has been lost, there should be a focus on those stressors which may have triggered the problem. If abuse is a potential issue, then extra measures are required and most particularly in ensuring the child's safety (see chapter 18).

In the child with a toilet phobia, treatment involves graded exposure and rewards.

Prognosis

Generally nearly all cases of uncomplicated encopresis resolve by adolescence, but a combined treatment approach leads to far speedier resolution. Attention to associated behaviour is also important.

Further reading

Clayden G, Agnasson U. *Constipation in childhood*. Oxford: Oxford University Press, 1991.

Fritz G, Rockney R. Enuresis. In: Kemberg P, Bemporad J, eds. *Handbook of child and adolescent psychiatry*, vol 2. *The grade-school child: development and syndromes*. New York: John Wiley, 1997:557–63.

White M, Epston D. *Narrative means to therapeutic ends*. New York: Norton, 1990.

12: Psychosis

Introduction

Psychosis is a frightening term and usually a terrifying experience for child and family. The nihilism and despair of previous eras carries over to the present day, even when the prognosis is better or, at worst, uncertain. What is often not appreciated by clinicians is how much it means for parents to be supported throughout the time of their child's psychosis and how much it means to the child or young person to be helped to make sense of what is happening.

Definition

Psychosis refers to a broad syndromal picture, a little like "cardiac failure" does in cardiology. It is not a diagnosis but a cluster of symptoms and signs, with a differential diagnosis. The essential feature of psychosis is a break down in the appreciation of reality.

A break down in the appreciation of reality

When reality appreciation of ideas and beliefs breaks down the process is referred to as delusional thinking. This is more than merely the holding of abnormal beliefs. Delusional thinking involves a disorder of conviction, which in its more extreme form assumes an unshakable quality.

When reality appreciation of perceptions breaks down, the process is referred to as hallucinosis and each experience as a hallucination.

When reality appreciation breaks down in the connectedness and coherence between one thought and the next the process is referred to as thought disorder.

The dimensional nature of experience

Each of these experiences is a matter of degree. For example a worry might become a preoccupation, a preoccupation may become an obsession, an obsession may become an overvalued idea, and an overvalued idea may become a delusion. Similarly, a visual stimulus may become an alluring image, which in turn may become an intrusive re-experiencing of a traumatic experience. These images may become illusions, which amplify and distort normal perceptions into objects of fear or desire. Illusions may become hallucinations. Normal meandering of thought may become poor concentration, which may become mental confusion, which in turn may become thought disorder.

Impairment of social response

Psychosis, then, is an impairment in reality appreciation in terms of belief, perception and the process of thought. But it is also an impairment in the sort of responses that emerge. Social responsiveness may be less discriminate, appropriate, or fine tuned. In the extreme, social blunting or bizarre behaviour may result. It can lead to both specific and generalised anxiety and mood changes. A transient sense of discomfort may become a persistent motor and mental restlessness and finally an inescapable agitation. In the extreme, the anxiety may be described as a pan-anxiety and the mood disturbance may be profound. In certain situations there is the emerging apprehension that something is about to happen of dire significance—referred to as apophany.

Differential diagnosis of psychosis in adolescence

- Psychotic depression
- Bipolar disorder (in particular bipolar I disorder, or what was formerly referred to as manic depressive illness)
- Organic psychosis including dementia, delirium, specific temporofrontal disorders, and substance induced disorders
- Schizophrenia and the schizophreniform disorders
- Brief psychotic disorder of childhood

- Benign hallucinosis
- Rare psychoses of childhood.

This chapter will concentrate on schizophrenia and the schizophreniform psychoses. The organic psychoses are dealt with in chapter 17 and psychotic depression and bipolar disorder are discussed in chapter 6. However, there are a number of rare disorders which are mentioned later.

Schizophrenic disorders

Introduction

The word schizophrenia evokes images of chronicity, raging insanity and, in the public mind, rapid alterations in personality with a relentless downhill course. For the most part these images are very inaccurate. Essentially schizophrenia is a psychosis for which no specific medical cause is identified that persists or recurs, and lacks a major disturbance of mood, other than blunting of affect. Where schizophrenia co-occurs with an affective picture the diagnosis schizoaffective disorder is used. While it can occur prepubertally, it is largely a disorder of late adolescence and early adulthood onset. Of course, chronicity and treatment unresponsiveness are real possibilities, but these need to be tempered with the improved prospects with early intervention programmes and more effective psychotropics.

Definitions

There are a number of different types of schizophrenia, but for the purposes of this chapter they are collectively referred to as schizophrenic disorders. These are characterised by fundamental distortions of thinking and perception, with blunted or inappropriate affect. Clear consciousness and intellectual capacity are ususally maintained. Common features include hallucinations, delusions, abnormalities or incoherence of thought, paucity of speech, social withdrawal, and apathy or restlessness. There are a number of subtypes:

- *Paranoid.* Marked by delusions referring to self. These may be persecutory or grandiose.
- *Catatonic.* Marked by motoric immobility, stupor, excessive purposeless motor activity, motiveless resistance to all instructions, and mutism.
- *Disorganised.* Gross thought disorder and facile affect.
- *Undifferentiated.* Most features are present and no one subtype predominates.
- *Residual.* A subsyndromal state following an acute episode.

Epidemiology

- Lifetime prevalence 1%
- Incidence of 0·01% per year
- More common in lower socioeconomic classes, especially the homeless, including homeless adolescents
- Very rare below age 7
- Uncommon below age 13, and with a male preponderance
- Peak time of presentation for males is 15–25 years and 25–35 in females, even though lifetime incidence is equal.

Aetiology and risk factors

Genetics

The lifetime risk of schizophrenia in the relatives of those with schizophrenia is shown in Table 12.1. Schizophrenia is most likely to be transmitted via multiple gene loci of small effect. Chromosones 6, 22, and 8 are of particular interest.

Family theories

There has been no support for the concept of "the schizophrenogenic mother", "the double bind hypothesis", or "the psychotic game" theory of schizophrenia. There is support for the view that increased numbers of relatives with schizotypal personalities, abnormal cognitive styles, and communication patterns predispose to schizophrenia. There is strong evidence that critical, emotionally overinvolved parents increase the chances of relapse.

Table 12.1 The lifetime risk of schizophrenia in the relatives of those with schizophrenia

Relationship	% with schizophrenia
Parent	5·6
Sibling	10·1
Sibling with one parent also affected	16·7
Children with one affected parent	12·8
Children with two affected parents	46·3
Uncles, aunts, nephews, and nieces	2·8
Grandchildren	3·7
General population	0·86

(With permission from Kendell RE, Zealley AK. *Companion to psychiatric studies*. Edinburgh: Churchill Livingstone, 1993.)

The neurodevelopmental hypothesis

Those who have very early onset are more likely (80%) to have a history of developmental impairment. It is likely that there are two groups of patients—the developmentally impaired group and the previously normal group.

Life events

Life events may precipitate but not cause schizophrenia.

The viral hypothesis

More people with schizophrenia are born in late winter and spring than at other times of the year. Exposure to viruses in the second and third trimester have been put forward as a possible cause of schizophrenia.

Neurochemical abnormalities

- The dopamine hypothesis proposes that hyperactivity of the dopaminergic system produces active symptoms.
- The serotonergic hypothesis is actually a modification of the dopamine hypothesis proposing that the ratio between

serotonergic activity and dopamine activity in the mesolimbic regions is critical.

- The excitatory amino acids glutamate and aspartate activity may be reduced in the limbic system.

Assessment and investigation

Practical hints:

- The withdrawn child raises the possibility of confusion with depressive disorders.
- The overactive child may lead to the diagnosis of attention deficit hyperactivity disorder (ADHD), the prescription of stimulants, and worsening of the psychosis.
- The dreamy child who has difficulty concentrating may be confused with attention deficit disorder.
- The overactive, confused talkative child with schizophrenia who is excited may appear manic.
- Perplexity, confusion and thought disorder may look like delirium.
- Bewilderment and high levels of arousal may look like an anxiety disorder but will generally not respond to reassurance or cognitive therapy.
- Social oddity in early primary school years raises the possibility of autistic spectrum disorders.
- School deterioration may raise the diagnosis of dementia.
- The teenager with a first episode of schizophrenia may be mistakenly thought to be taking marijuana or other illicit substances. A drug screen may be helpful.
- Inappropriate sexual behaviour and delusions about HIV may raise the issue of sexual abuse quite unnecessarily.
- If in doubt whether the child has a mood disorder with psychosis (psychotic depression or mania) or schizophrenia disorder with secondary mood disorder consider the following:

  - If acute containment is required treat as if schizophrenia but keep open to the possibility of depression or mania.
  - If there is no immediate issue of containment treat as if an affective disorder but keep open to the possibility of schizophrenia.

- If it remains unclear over time opt for affective disorder since this has the better prognosis and response to treatment. It is better to err on the side of optimism and greater treatment options.
- If there are marked personal eccentricities consider Asperger's disorder as an alternative or comorbid disorder.
- If the age of onset is between 3 and 7 years consider disintegrative disorder or dementia.
- If hallucinations are visual, illusions are prominent, sleep cycle reversal is present and confusion is marked, consider an organic psychosis, particularly drug induced psychosis. Fine tremor, wide eyes, tactile and visual hallucinations and a tachycardia suggest a drug induced psychosis in general and anticholinergic psychosis in particular.
- The younger the child the more likely are confusion and hallucinations to feature. The older the child the more likely are paranoid delusions to predominate.
- When children and young people begin to become psychotic they may become anxious, depressed, or preoccupied about worries from the past or present. When they are recovering they may well experience the same phenomena. These experiences may indicate a less grave diagnosis.
- As with the affective psychoses, in the acute phase of the illness issues erupt from the inner life of the child and adolescent like lava from a volcano. It is important not to put too much aetiological weight on these outpourings but rather observe the process rather than the content of what is happening.
- The general tendency in adolescence is to overdiagnose schizophrenia and underdiagnose bipolar disorder.
- Substance abuse must always be considered as a symptom, a precipitant, and a complication, and just occasionally as a cause of the young person's condition.
- Schizophrenia-like behaviour is sometimes considered to be fabricated. Occasionally the young person with schizophrenia will even claim this to be the case. However it is in fact very hard to sustain psychotic behaviour willfully. It is very unusual for those who are truly deceitful and lying to acknowledge it.
- Premorbid function—the earlier the onset the more likely there is to have been a history of odd, anxious behaviour or antisocial tendencies. In fact almost any picture might be

Table 12.2 Negative and positive symptoms in the presentation of schizophrenia

Positive symptoms	Negative symptoms
Hallucinations	Poverty of affect
Delusions	Poverty of speech
Thought disorder	Poverty of motivation
Disorganised behaviour	Disexecutive syndrome (i.e. difficulty in planning, deciding and making judgements)

present! There is likely to have been premorbid abnormal behaviour in up to 50%. In the rest, the presentation is sudden.

Investigation involves a urinary drug screen, exclusion of medication induced causes (for example antihistamines, anticholinergic drugs, and stimulants in high dose), review for possible causes of dementia (mitochondrial, viral, inflammatory, seizure related, neurodegenerative, and space occupying) and delirium (encephalitis and sleep disorders).

Clinical presentation

The clinical presentation of schizophrenia varies along a range of different dimensions, described below.

The symptom–deficit dimension

In general the more acute the picture the more "positive" are the symptoms and the more chronic the picture the more "negative" are the symptoms (Table 12.2).

The acute–insidious dimension

Most clinicians recognise four phases:

1. Prodromal
2. Acute
3. Convalescent
4. Residual.

Patients may present in any of these phases even though the acute phase is more likely.

Organised–disorganised thought dimension

Highly systematised delusional presentations, especially of a paranoid child or adolescent, will look very different from the vague or incoherent ramblings.

Active–passive or motor dimension

Catatonia may present as complete motor immobility or acute overactive excitement.

It is clear that there is often a convergence of positive symptoms, acuteness of onset, later onset, organisation of thought, and motor activity on the one hand, and negative symptoms, insidious onset, disorganised thought, and passivity on the other. However, various combinations of presentation at different times of the illness are possible.

Treatment

This must be comprehensive.

Antipsychotic medication

Antipsychotic medication is the mainstay of treatment. In the young, extrapyramidal side effects are the rule rather than the exception, especially in the acute dystonias. Therefore, the atypical antipsychotics are the first line treatment rather than second line antipsychotics. Risperidone and olanzapine are the most widely available and least problematic. Furthermore, there is evidence that olanzapine is helpful for the negative symptoms of schizophrenia. These produce sedation particularly over the first 3–5 days. They begin to take effect over 3–6 weeks and produce their maximal effect over 3–6 months continuing to give improvement in longer term cases up to 1 year. The very early onset group does not respond as well to antipsychotic medication and the school or residential setting will be the most critical component of treatment.

Agitation must be treated vigorously. Benzodiazapines are helpful when insomnia is prominent and the agitation is not fully assuaged by the antipsychotics. Short term adjunctive use of a low potency typical antipsychotic such as thioridazine may help.

Family therapy

- The family dynamics are not explored in the acute phase of the psychosis, as this may aggravate the problem.
- Educational approaches are proven to be helpful. These focus on:
  - the nature of schizophrenia—what it is and it is not
  - lowering emotional intensity
  - enhancing parental support
  - lowering criticism
  - ensuring a clear structure for each day
  - reducing environmental demand
  - informing others of what is helpful and reasonable
  - encouraging adherence to medication
  - supporting low short term expectations and realistic but solid long term expectations.
- Educating the young person:
  - in the acute phase—reassurance, distress reduction, reality orientation
  - in the longer term explaining about the nature of illness.

Cognitive behaviour therapy

Medication is not always able to abolish troubling thoughts, hallucinations, and difficulties in coping. Cognitive techniques may help with these (see chapter 24).

Course and prognosis

Complications

- Self neglect.
- Poor nutrition.
- Isolation and loneliness—stigma, misunderstanding and fear of others may be pervasive.

- Increased accidents. These may be in response to hallucinations or delusions.
- Violence. This is rare but gains media attention. Young people with schizophrenia do not commit most of the violence that does occur. When violence does occur in schizophrenia, it mostly occurs out of fearful delusions. Patients with schizophrenia are 100 times more likely to commit suicide than homocide.
- Despair. This may be greater than in the affective disorders and sometimes is reality based. Companionship, access to care, and sympathetic institutional structures reduce the isolation of despair.
- Failure to fulfil academic and social expectations.
- Loss of motivation, decision making, forward planning, and selective attention.
- Homelessness.
- Suicide occurs in about 10%. Most occur in the first 10 years of the disorder and males are greater (twofold) than females.

There is a great degree of variability in course and prognosis. Blanket pessimism is unjustified. A relentless downhill course with each episode over the first 5 years, without return to normality, occurs in about a third of patients. About 10% will suffer all their impairment as a result of the first episode. They may have further episodes but there will be no further reduction in social functioning. Over 50% will have little residual social impairment. About 20% will have one episode only with no ongoing impairment. There is a tendency toward clinical improvement after the middle decades of life.

Brief psychotic disorder

This is an uncommon phenomenon in which children and adolescents may have short-lived delusions, hallucinations, thought disorder with incoherence of speech and disorganised or catatonic behaviour. They are frequently confused, agitated, and in turmoil. They are at particular risk of suicide. Such features were previously thought to be a response to stress and were labelled brief reactive psychoses. However, it is now known that they may occur without stressors and, in adulthood, in the postpartum period. It is likely that at least some are related to the mood disorders especially if they are recurrent. Others may go on to develop schizophreniform disorders, but for many they never recur.

Benign hallucinosis of childhood

The experience of hallucinations in the absence of delusion, thought disorder, behavioural control or impaired peer relations is uncommon in childhood and adolescence. It often presents in articulate, well educated children; perhaps they are able to communicate their concerns to parents who are aware of the potential gravity of hallucinations. Complex partial seizures, viral infections, head injury, and drug toxicity need to be excluded. The condition is usually self-remitting, occasionally recurrent, and disappears promptly with a short course of low dose atypical antipsychotics. There is no evidence at this stage that these children go on to develop longer term psychotic disorders.

Rare psychoses in children and adolescents

Kleine–Levin syndrom

This syndrome has recurrent episodes of hypersomnia, hyperphagia, confusion and psychotic symptoms, which initially appear to be a delirium but may evolve into a bipolar disorder. There is generally full recovery between episodes. It was thought to only occur in boys but is increasingly seen in girls. CSF analysis may reveal low serotonin breakdown products (5OH indoleacetic acid).

Peripubertal psychosis

This may appear to be like Kleine–Levin or schizophrenia but again is associated with marked affectivity, recurrence, and full interepisodic recovery.

Menstrually related hypersomnia

These young girls have psychotic episodes just prior to and in association with menarche often on a monthly basis, with full recovery after 5–10 days. Again these often evolve into an affective disorder. They respond to antipsychotics and mood stabilisers, or occasionally to oestrogen preparations.

Viral induced psychosis

Children and young people may have subclinical viral infections (in the sense that very little evidence of the viral illness is present) involving the CNS and, instead of frank encephalitis with neurological disorder, have psychiatric manifestations. CSF reveals raised titres for neurotoxic viruses such as herpes and coxsackie. They respond to antipsychotics and, occasionally, antiviral agents. The children may be left with mild to moderate intellectual impairment.

Delirium with psychosis

See chapter 17.

Conclusion

Psychosis in childhood and adolescence is serious and requires high quality and youth friendly services. A family based approach is essential if support is to be given and complications are to be reduced. These disorders are among the most frightening and distressing in medicine and an appreciation of the uncertainty, fears and misunderstandings faced by patients and their families is essential. The armamentarium at our disposal is immeasurably greater than at any previous time in history. Despite this the prognosis for the very early onset group needs to be improved and the burden of care remains considerable. In the acute phases agitation needs to receive a higher priority for treatment and in the chronic phases motivation requires more attention.

Further reading

Fuller-Torrey E. *Surviving schizophrenia: a family manual.* New York: Basic Books, 2001.

Fuller-Torrey E, Bowler A, Taylor EH, Gottesmann I. *Schizophrenia and manic depressive disorder.* New York: Basic Books, 1994.

Werry JS. Childhood schizophrenia. In: Volkmar FR, ed. *Psychoses and pervasive developmental disorders in childhood and adolescence.* Washington: American Psychiatric Press and American Academy of Child and Adolescent Psychiatry, 1996:1–8.

13: Somatisation

Introduction

Somatisation is the communication of emotional distress, troubled relationships and personal predicaments through bodily symptoms. The symptoms suggest an underlying medical condition but no organic disease can be found to account for them, nor are the symptoms under conscious control.

Aetiology

This tends to be multifactorial with family factors being particularly relevant. Not only are family members more likely to present with somatic complaints, but they are also more likely to have a chronic physical illness or disability and thus probably provide a model for the patient's symptoms. Other family factors include marital disharmony, undue expectations of achievement, high levels of depression or anxiety, disorganisation, and substance misuse.

Symptoms may be reinforced by excess attention, either in the form of overinvestigation or parental overconcern, or by consequent avoidance of situations perceived by the child to be difficult or distressing.

Trauma, including all forms of abuse, may give rise to somatisation, as may altered mood states such as depresson and anxiety.

Epidemiology

Single somatic symptoms, in particular abdominal pain, headaches, low energy, dizziness, nausea, vomiting and limb pains are common, particularly in girls. However, in the main they do not reach the criteria for somatisation disorder as they are generally monosymptomatic. There appears to be a developmental sequence in the type of symptoms displayed.

The prepubertal child experiences affective distress as recurrent abdominal pain (this symptom peaking at age 9 years) and headaches (peaking at age 12 years). With increasing age, limb pain, aching muscles, fatigue and neurological symptoms become more prominent. Overall, polysymptomatic somatisation becomes more common as age increases.

Clinical features

The most common forms of somatisation are: (a) recurrent abdominal pain; (b) other sites of pain; (c) fatigue; and (d) conversion symptoms. Before dealing with each in turn it should be emphasised that there is commonly overlap between them and comorbidity is probably more common than not.

Recurrent abdominal pain

Recurrent abdominal pain (RAP) affects between 10% and 20% of school aged children at some time in their childhood and is one of the most common presenting symptoms. It may occur as often as every day or far less frequently. It may be limited to school days or coincide with upsetting events in the home, such as parental conflict, or other specific situations. RAP is sometimes associated with headaches, nausea, vomiting, or limb pain. It can of course be superimposed upon organic disease such as constipation, irritable bowel syndrome, appendicitis, urinary tract infection, mesenteric adenitis, inflammatory bowel disorders, gastro-oesophageal reflux, gastritis, enterobacter pylori, small bowel dysmotility, or carbohydrate malabsorption. A full history and examination is therefore imperative. However in the vast majority of cases no organic cause is found and there is usually some underlying emotional stressor.

Pains in other sites

These are also relatively common in childhood. They may be located in the limbs, joints, muscles, head, or chest. The child may often deny any worries or distress other than the pain. Precipitants seem strangely absent and often contributing factors do not become evident until treatment is in progress. A careful exploration should be made to exclude an organic cause as either a complete or partial explanation for the pain. In the physical examination inconsistencies between the presentation and knowledge of anatomical pathways should be noted. Inconsistency is not pathognomonic of psychological disorder but it may be suggestive.

In general physical abnormalities found tend to result from inactivity due to pain, for example muscle wasting, reduced flexibility, and contractures. However it is important to exclude the possibility of organic causes for headache such as the need for glasses, migraine, tumours, and cerebral infections. Conditions that need consideration in joint and limb pains include arthritis, trauma, inflammatory processes, and infections. Possible causes of chest pain include infections and reflux oesophagitis.

Pains can masquerade depression and anxiety and may occur alongside other forms of somatisation, such as fatigue and conversion disorder (see below).

Fatigue

The experience of considerable fatigue with no obvious organic explanation appears to be an increasingly common symptom in childhood. Fatigue as an isolated symptom may occur but more commonly it is associated with other features. There has been enormous controversy as to whether there is an underlying but undiagnosed organic condition in many such cases. The term "ME" (myalgic encephalitis) is often used to account for a range of symptoms which have fatigue as their central core. Other features include a range of pains, loss of appetite, weakness, dizziness, and other sensory or motor disturbances. There is sometimes an obvious organic precipitant such as a viral infection or some form of trauma, which is then given not only causal significance but also is considered to be maintaining the disorder. In general organic investigation fails to reveal any obvious disease and the abnormal findings are usually a result of weight loss, inactivity, or muscle wasting.

More recently the term chronic fatigue syndrome (CFS) has gained acceptance. Its advantage is that it simply describes the condition without making assumptions as to aetiology or pathological processes. The term "ME" assumes a pathophysiological process within the muscles and brain, for which there is virtually no evidence.

In reality it is very likely that the symptom of fatigue is a feature of a continuum of conditions. Without doubt fatigue occurs in a wide range of organic conditions and is also a common symptom in depression, anxiety, and other emotional disorders. Whilst it is a common feature of any acute illness, it usually resolves with the illness. However in some cases it persists for no obvious reason. Not uncommonly underlying psychological factors such as school, peer-group or family related stresses are in due course uncovered. In any event the resulting inactivity may contribute to a vicious cycle. An initial infection or trauma gives rise to fatigue, which prevents activity, which in turn leads to altered mood and lowered morale, further inactivity, and eventually loss of fitness and muscle weakness.

The child's deterioration and inability to participate in normal daily activity reinforces the conviction that there must be a underlying organic cause. The wise clinician will always have borne this possibility in mind, indeed should never discount it, but rarely is an organic explanation found.

Conversion symptoms

These are manifested by a motor or sensory deficit without organic explanation.

Motor symptoms include seizure-like activity, abnormal gait, movements or coordination, and weakness or paralysis. Any body part can be affected including the vocal cords, resulting in mutism or vocal cord dysfunction. Vocal cord dysfunction can lead to clinical symptoms that are similar to asthma but unresponsive to pharmacotherapy, and in extreme cases can lead to intubation and ventilation.

Sensory disturbances most commonly affect the extremities and are often associated with motor dysfunction. The site and distribution of the disturbance will often not relate to any anatomical pathway but correlate with the patient's ideas of nerve distribution such as a glove and stocking pattern. Symptoms can also include loss of any sensation including hearing and vision.

Clues to a diagnosis of conversion are inconsistencies such as loss of vision but not bumping into objects, normal neurological examination, and normal investigations. On physical examination abnormalities will often not correspond to a neuroanatomical explanation for the presentation. However, if there is a model upon which the disorder is based and the imitation is accurate it may follow a roughly anatomical distribution. Not uncommonly the child appears to have less concern about the problem than would be expected, a reaction sometimes described as "belle indifference".

As with all somatisation symptoms conversion may mask organic disease as well as anxiety, depression, substance abuse, post-traumatic stress disorder, factitious disorder, and malingering. It is paramount as mentioned earlier to exclude the main possible neurological and medical conditions that could give rise to the symptoms that are presented. Furthermore, even when a conversion disorder has been diagnosed, the possibility of a comorbid medical diagnosis should not be forgotten, including multiple sclerosis and other muscle and neurological disorders.

Management

As with most conditions this must be comprehensive and should include parental counselling, physical rehabilitation, cognitive behavioural therapy, and in some cases medication.

The parental counselling should include as clear as possible an explanation of the condition, explaining how the conclusion has been reached. It is helpful to explain the ways in which stress can give rise to physical symptoms and to give everyday examples in adult life, such as tension headaches. When parents are resistant to such explanations a confrontational approach should be avoided; rather it is better to discuss with them what they think might be wrong and how this could be investigated. It is important that a physician remains involved, even if the charge of the case is handed on to a mental health care worker. In this way the parents do not feel that they are not being taken seriously, that they have been "dumped" onto someone else, that they are "crazy", or that they are being blamed for their child's problems. In addition, the possibility of organic disease is not being dismissed whilst attempts are made to help overcome the underlying problems.

If there is resistance to psychological input a joint meeting between parent, child, paediatrician and mental health worker may help. Children and parents need to feel they have been heard, understood, respected, and believed. The paediatrician can explain what is not wrong and how the conclusions have been reached. It should be possible to describe a model of the illness that is acceptable to all parties, such as "pain makes you feel depressed and irritable which makes the pain harder to live with". This can be aided by using the family's words and an optimistic approach usually aids the process.

Finding "face savers" is important. This is often best achieved either by physical rehabilitation or medication. Physiotherapy and graded mobilisation can be particularly useful for fatigue and motor deficits. They prevent muscle weakness and promote mobility. For motor deficits the focus can initially be on non-affected parts (what is well keep well) and passive activity, followed by a very gradual increase in activity of the affected parts. Hydrotherapy is particularly helpful because of the absence of weight bearing and its potential for saving face. Furthermore it can be made enjoyable. In fatigue states graded mobilisation can be presented like a fitness training programme, as would be used by anyone trying to gain strength and fitness. Again hydrotherapy is valuable.

Cognitive behavioural therapy (see chapter 24) is often helpful in giving the child a means of mastering the physical symptoms and tackling any underlying concerns.

Medication may be of value in treating underlying anxiety or depression. It is reasonable to provide short term analgesia, tricyclic antidepressants, carbamazepine or gabapentin for pain.

In summary, early intervention is important and a graded approach with specific but low key steps is most likely to succeed. The focus should be on what the child can rather than cannot do.

Although up to a quarter of children with RAP may continue to have abdominal pain or migraine in adult life, the prognosis for somatisation is usually reasonable providing appropriate treatment is available and utilised. Resistance to treatment usually worsens the outlook and may lead to chronicity.

Conclusion

There are few areas of medicine or psychology that are so prone to misunderstanding between patients, their parents and clinicians as somatisation. However, providing the clinician adopts a comprehensive, sympathetic and non-confrontational approach, it is generally possible to help children and their parents to full recovery.

Further reading

Apley J, McKeith R, Meadow R. *The child and his symptoms: a comprehensive approach*, 3rd edn. Oxford: Blackwell, 1978.

Brazier DK, Venning HE. Conversion disorder in adolescents: a practical approach to rehabilitation. *British Journal of Rheumatology* 1997;**36**:594–8.

Campo J, Fritsch S. Somatization in children and adolescents. *Journal of the American Academy of Child and Adolsecent Psychiatry* 1994;**33**:1223–5.

De Maso D, Beasley P. The somatoform disorders. In: Klykylo W, Kay J, Rube D, eds. *Clinical child psychiatry*, 1st edn. Pennsylvania: WB Saunders, 1998; 429–444.

Fritz GK, Fritsch S, Hagino O. Somatoform disorders in children and adolescents: a review of the past 10 years. *Journal American Academy of Child and Adolescent Psychiatry* 1997;**36**:1329–39.

Gooch JL, Wolcott R, Speed J. Behavioural management of conversion disorder in children. *Archives of Physical Medicine and Rehabilitation* 1997;**78**:264–8.

Pilowsky I. *Abnormal illness behaviour*. Chichester: Wiley, 1997.

14: Psychiatric aspects of the medically ill child

Introduction

This chapter focuses on the emotional and behavioural needs of children with medical illnesses together with the response and strain that exist within the family caring for the ill child.

With medical advances children are making complete recoveries from previously fatal illnesses such as leukaemia, are living longer with chronic illnesses such as cystic fibrosis and HIV, and technological advances are presenting new opportunities for organ failure such as transplantation. Psychiatric sequelae in these situations are common, requiring comprehensive care in liaison with psychiatric services.

First the epidemiology of psychiatric disturbances will be discussed, followed by issues common to chronic medical illnesses and approaches to the assessment. Subsequently, issues particular to specific illnesses will be described.

Epidemiology

About 15–20% of children will have a chronic illness with 10% of them (approximately 2% of all children) suffering from a severe illness that effects growth, development, access to education and social needs. These include illnesses such as cystic fibrosis, sickle cell anaemia, arthritis, HIV infection, spina bifida, diabetes, and asthma. By and large the majority of children cope well with the stress related to the illness and the treatment. However psychiatric disturbance occurs in between 20% and 30% of those with a medical illness, with figures of up to 50% being noted for those with disfiguring features or a neurological component.

Psychological aspects of medical illness

When considering a child with a medical illness the main focus should be on the interactions between the child, the illness, the family, and extrafamilial factors—"the illness network". Though the elements of the network will be considered separately, this delineation is artificial with each component having a reciprocal impact on the other.

The illness and the child

The response to the illness can sometimes be more handicapping than the actual illness. Illness will have an impact on all domains of the child's life—physical, social, and psychological—which in turn can act to perpetuate or aggravate the illness. For instance, depression and anger in response to an illness such as cystic fibrosis can result in refusal to do the physiotherapy, reduction in food intake with loss of weight, and subsequent worsening of illness.

Important factors that determine adjustment to an illness include:

- *Aspects of the illness.* These include the severity, chronicity, its course and whether it relapses or remits, the presence of constant discomfort, how generalised it is, and the intrusiveness and demands of the treatment regimen.
- *Constraints resulting from illness.* For example, the child being unable to engage with athletic activities or mix with his/her peer group.
- *Age of the child.* Different stresses will have a differential impact depending on the developmental stage of the child. In infancy illness may affect attachment and developmental milestones such as autonomy and mobility. After 5 years there will be a greater impact on educational progress, athletic activities, and achievement. In adolescence social adjustment, individual identity, independence from the family, and poor adherence to treatment become more of an issue. Prolonged separation will have a particular negative impact between the ages of 6 months and 3 years.

- *Personality features.* A child who is more adaptable to new situations and responds well to change will fair better. By contrast, a child who from early life has been difficult to soothe with an insecure attachment relationship has an increased risk for poor outcome.
- *Intellectual capacity.* Children who are brighter will generally have better coping skills.

The child can be affected by the illness in many ways with cognitive, emotional, behavioural and somatic responses. These responses, though considered individually, interact with each other.

Cognitive style

Response to the illness can lie anywhere along the spectrum of overacceptance to denial and may fluctuate with time. Both extremes can result in problems, with the parents often adopting similar attitudes. A child who displays overacceptance may be susceptible to the illness taking over, overshadowing all aspects of life, and resulting in high levels of anxiety about the slightest symptom. By contrast, denial can result in ignoring symptoms and warning signs, poor adherence to treatment, and engaging in activities which may precipitate worsening of the illness.

Children may have fantasies and myths about the cause and prognosis of their disease, such as the illness being punishment for a misdemeanour. These fantasies need to be elicited and replaced by what is often the less frightening reality.

Emotional response

At the time of the diagnosis the child and family may proceed through a response similar to a bereavement reaction with shock, denial, anger, acceptance, and adjustment. This pattern of response may be repeated at times of disease relapse. These are all normal responses to a serious illness, so long as the child proceeds through the phases. When sadness deepens to depression with excessive unprecipitated crying, withdrawal, reduced food intake, irritability, inactivity, and sleep disturbances, intervention is necessary. Anxiety disorders have also been noted at increased rates.

The extent to which a child expresses feelings will depend on both his/her own and the family's style of emotional expression. In families who find it hard to tolerate negative emotions help may be needed in identifying and expressing emotions.

The child's self-esteem and body image may be affected by the illness, and these can be intensified or even exacerbated by a faulty cognitive self-appraisal.

Behavioural response

The behavioural response will depend on age with regression, for example losing recently established milestones such as dryness at night being a common sequel to illness.

In infancy crying and feeding problems may occur, whilst the toddler may become hyperactive as well as displaying sleep and feeding disturbances. Subsequently difficulties with toileting, academic performance and peer relationships predominate.

Another problem that may be encountered is poor adherence to treatment. Reasons for this are multifold and include:

- Denial of the illness
- Failure to fully understand the instructions or need for treatment
- Anxieties about the treatment
- Belief that the treatment will not work
- Past history of negative experiences of treatment
- Disorganised families
- Initial clinical improvement
- Unpleasant or intolerable side effects
- Peer group pressure
- The burdens, financial, practical, social, and psychological, of adherence
- Feelings of hopelessness or a desire to die
- A psychiatric illness, for example depression.

Somatic responses

The child may respond to anxiety and distress in somatic ways with a heightened awareness and sensitivity to bodily symptoms, for instance in the form of recurrent abdominal pain.

The family and the illness

The illness can have detrimental effects on the family and family dysfunction can aggravate the illness.

The effect of the illness on the family

Some families are united by the adversity whilst others respond with increasing disharmony. Mothers are more likely than fathers to respond with distress and depressive symptoms, though all family members are affected emotionally, financially, and physically.

Parental care may involve the physical burden of daily physiotherapy and lifting the patient from one setting to another. Financial burdens may include special diets, equipment, time off work, and transportation costs. Psychiatric morbidity has been found to be greater in parents of children with chronic illness than their healthy counterparts.

As for the child, the parental response may lie anywhere along the spectrum of denial to overinvolvement. In families where the parents are overinvolved the child may be so overprotected that the parents are unable to allow the child to experience the normal aspects of life or to appropriately discipline them.

Siblings can be affected in a number of ways. They can be relatively neglected as a result of the increased amount of time invested in the sick child, or they might feel overburdened with responsibility for care of the sibling, or lose friendships because of stigma of the illness.

The effect of the family on the illness

Family dysfunction can precipitate or maintain a disease whilst specific healthy factors can improve its prognosis. These include a good marriage, an optimal realistic attitude, satisfactory adaptation, stability, warmth, cohesion, and good parental communication. Factors associated with a poor outcome include marital disharmony, rigid or disorganised families, overprotective or denying families, and poor communication. Guilt can also influence the ability of the family to support the medical plan. This can arise from feelings of responsibility for the child developing the illness, for example following a car accident, or in the case of hereditary diseases.

Extrafamilial factors

Factors lying outside of the family that can influence the illness network include the school, healthcare workers, peers, neighbours, and extended families. As part of the normal process of adjustment and grief following a diagnosis anger may be displaced on to others. This can include healthcare workers and may result in the worker feeling criticised, angry, or inadequate.

Assessment

Assessment will need to be guided by the problems being presented, the child's developmental status, and the nature of the illness. Clinicians generally underdetect behavioural problems in such children.

Key topics that need to be covered are described below.

Screening for psychopathology

This includes:

- The child's and family reaction to the illness, distress and pain, coping strategies, and communication styles.
- Any risk factors and vulnerabilities in the child or environment.

Screening instruments can be used to enhance recognition, for example the child behaviour checklist, but they have reduced efficacy in the medically ill child.

Cognitive assessment

The cognitive assessment is important for children with central nervous system involvement and those suffering from the secondary effects of stress or systemic disease. An impaired cognitive state influences problem solving ability and coping. Instruments that can be used include:

• Stanford-Binet intelligence test, fourth edition
• Weschler tests
• Leiter-R for language deficits.

Assessment of social functioning and quality of life

An assessment of social confidence and peer relationships is important because when compromised they are risk factors for behavioural problems.

Assessment of quality of life may best be evaluated using both generic[1] and disease specific questionnaires (for example, paediatric cancer,[2] spina bifida,[3] and asthma[4]).

These instruments should evaluate social, physical and emotional functioning alongside disease and treatment related symptoms.

Hope is essential for medically ill children and those involved in their care, and helps to maintain treatment adherence. However this needs to be balanced with realism about the medical risks involved. Snyder *et al.*[5] have developed a scale which assesses hope.

The psychiatric aspects of specific illnesses

Asthma

Psychological factors probably play a role in precipitating and increasing the severity of individual attacks alongside other triggers such as immunological, infectious and physiological.

Children with asthma are twice as likely to suffer emotional disturbance compared to healthy children, especially those who develop it before the age of 3. The problems include sleep disturbance, depressed mood, and anxiety. The treatments for asthma, such as corticosteroids and salbutamol, can in their own right precipitate behavioural disturbances.

When children die from asthma, depression, denial, emotional triggers for attacks and unsupportive families are found to be more frequent concomitants than any physical elements.

Cystic fibrosis

With advances in management there has been a significant increase in life expectancy in children with cystic fibrosis. Genetic advances have allowed identification of individuals prenatally with all the surrounding controversy.

The severity of cystic fibrosis is the main predictor of psychiatric disturbance, with eating difficulties, poor adherence and anxiety about the shortened life span being the particular concerns in these children.

Leukaemia

Leukaemia is the commonest childhood malignancy. The development of rigorous treatment regimens have increased 5 year survival to over 50%. However some of the treatments involve direct effects of brain function through cranial irradiation, may be painful, and leave the child and family in a persisting state of uncertainty. It is therefore not surprising that there is an increased risk of psychiatric morbidity.

Particular times of vulnerability occur around the time of diagnosis, during active treatment, and following the consequences of treatment. Treatment heralds pain, adverse side effects including hair loss, nausea, and infection. During this time approximately one third will have symptoms of anxiety, sadness, and clinging behaviour. Cranial irradiation can result in neuropsychological deficits including short term memory loss, inattention, and cerebral atrophy. Other complications of treatment include impaired growth, organ failure, and secondary malignancy. Improved adaptation is associated with open communication between family members and healthcare professionals and good peer support.

Skin disorders

Approximately one third of children with skin disorders have associated emotional problems. Causality is bidirectional. Disfiguring conditions such as eczema and vitiligo lead to lowered self-esteem and mood changes, whilst emotional distress can potentiate itching, hair pulling, and excoriation.

Psychological effects of skin disorders

Atopic dermatitis is predominantly a condition of early childhood with many having complete remission in the first few years. It therefore has few long term implications but may herald future atopic disorders such as allergic rhinitis and asthma. Eczema, especially when involving visible parts of the body, may result in rejection by parents and peers who may fear contracting the disorder. The importance of emotional support and physical contact needs to be emphasised. Eliciting the help of previously affected family members may help when stressing the good long term prognosis.

Skin disorders reflective of psychological disorders

Relentless excoriation can result from psychological disturbances. This includes anxiety disorder, obsessive compulsive disorder, attention deficit hyperactivity disorder, and Tourettes's syndrome. Though the presentation tends to be dermatological, the underlying psychological disorder must be identified. Rauch et al.[6] have developed a checklist for identifying which children may require psychological referral.

Dermatitis artifacta involves self-infliction of skin lesions, often as a reaction to stress. Alternatively, a parent may produce the lesion (see fabricated or induced illness by carer—chapter 18), for example by shaving the child's head and saying the hair loss followed chemotherapy.

Diabetes

Living with diabetes in childhood requires adherence to an intrusive treatment regimen, including a strict diet, urine and blood testing for glucose control, and the administration of insulin injections. Teenagers in particular find this restriction on lifestyle at a time when they are experiencing conflicts with control and autonomy particularly demanding. Results of studies on psychiatric morbidity and diabetes have been conflicting, though the consensus is that diabetic teenagers are more at risk for psychological disturbances than their healthy counterparts.

As a result of the generally later onset, early parent–child attachment is rarely disrupted. However, both the restriction the illness places on the child and the stress incurred in managing the disorder for both the child and family can result in depression, anxiety and adjustment disorder in the child and family dysfunction in the vulnerable family.

A relationship has been found between low serum glucose and triglyceride levels in stressed diabetic adolescents, and in dysfunctional families elevated glycosylated haemoglobin has been noted.

Poor diabetic control has been correlated with the presence of a psychiatric illness, reading difficulties and psychosocial adversity, and in those with onset prior to 5 years, cognitive difficulties have been found even when only mild hyperglycaemia had occurred.

Epilepsy

Epilepsy is associated with a particularly high rate of psychiatric comorbidity, with figures of around 30%. Possible reasons include:

- *The nature of the underlying pathology.* The origin of the brain dysfunction can determine the type of psychiatric problem. For example, in temporal lobe seizures psychosis, hyperkinetic syndrome and rage tends to occur relatively frequently. Behavioural problems occur particularly in boys, and when there is an early onset of seizures. Treatment-resistant seizures are more strongly associated with psychiatric and behavioural sequelae than those that are well controlled. In tuberous sclerosis the behavioural difficulties may pre-date the epilepsy. Some syndromes (for example Lennox–Gastaut) are associated with severe developmental regression.

- *Direct effect of the seizure.* Depression, psychosis and reduced cognitive performance can all be related to the ictal event.
- *Result of treatment.* Anticonvulsants can cause a wide range of psychiatric morbidity, and this is shown in detail in Box 14.1.
- *Psychosocial factors.* These include stigmatisation, subjective feelings of lack of control, and reduced expectations from parents of academic potential. Observers of seizures may fear the child had gone mad or that death is imminent. The education of teachers, peers, siblings and family members is paramount.

It is important to remember that often the consequences of the fits have a greater negative effect on the child's and family's lives than the seizure themselves. Therefore monitoring seizure rate as the only measure of outcome may be doing a disservice to the family. In addition, alleviating some of the psychiatric problems may well reduce both the frequency and severity of the fits.

Cerebral palsy

There is a fivefold increased risk of psychiatric morbidity in those with cerebral palsy approximating to about 50% of sufferers. In the main the full range of disorders are seen, but in those with comorbid mental retardation, overactivity and autistic features are overrepresented.

Similar to epilepsy, contributing factors include:

- An underlying brain dysfunction
- Cognitive impairment
- Specific reading retardation increasing the risk of psychiatric problems
- Psychosocial factors such as reduced self-esteem and self-image, stigmatisation, bullying, and rejection by peers
- Family dysfunction.

The situation will be compounded by associated sensory deficits, epilepsy, and learning disorder, all increasing the risk of psychiatric morbidity.

Box 14.1 Psychiatric morbidity resulting from anticonvulsants

- Barbiturates

  - hyperactivity
  - aggression
  - learning deficits
  - cognitive impairment
  - depression

- Benzodiazepines

  - aggression
  - depression
  - disinhibition
  - irritability
  - cognitive impairment

- Carbamazepine

  - depression
  - irritability
  - psychosis (though it has antimanic and antidepressant qualities)

- Ethosuximide

  - psychosis, personality change
  - irritability

- Gabapentin

  - aggression
  - hyperactivity

- Phenytoin

  - affective disorder
  - confusion
  - cognitive impairment
  - progressive encephalopathy
  - hyperactivity and rage

- Sodium valproate

  - progressive encephalopathy
  - depression

- Vigabatrin

  - depression
  - psychosis

Cerebral tumours

Brain tumours are rare although the second most common childhood malignancy. Two thirds tend to be located in the subtentorial region and a small minority are metastatic secondaries. Presentation depends on the location of the tumour and rapidity of growth.

Psychological presentations are non-specific such as irritability and aggression with physical symptoms such as headache, vomiting, gait disturbance, fits and cranial nerve involvement the more prominent presenting features.

Those with brainstem involvement, particularly pontine tumours, may show marked behavioural disturbances that can lead to misdiagnosis. These include lethargy, apathy, aggression, hyperactivity, impaired concentration, bed wetting, and disruption of sleep. Treatment, be it surgery or irradiation, can result in psychiatric morbidity. Sequelae include specific learning disability, intellectual decline, and non-specific psychiatric problems such as aggression.

Hearing impairment

Approximately 0·4% of children suffer from moderate to profound hearing impairment of congenital or acquired forms. Transitory hearing impairment from acute ear infections is extremely common. A minority of these suffer from persisting mild to moderate hearing loss. The vast majority of deaf children are born to hearing parents. For the family the impact of confirmation of diagnosis is emotionally overwhelming and resembles the bereavement reaction.

Psychiatric morbidity occurs in between 25% and 50%, with anxiety disorders predominating. Communication difficulties are obviously common and hearing parents are forced to adjust to different means of communication and management with consequent frustration, anger, and depression. Other problems include social immaturity, reduced opportunities to socialise, increased pressure to achieve, and limited imaginary play. These can result in a feeling of social isolation and difficulties in forming interpersonal relationships.

The impact on intellectual functioning is variable. However there is generally a shorter short term memory span with greater reliance on visual–spatial short term coding.

Visual impairment

About six children in every thousand are partially sighted or blind. Common causes include hereditary retinopathies, cortical blindness, congenital anomalies, cataracts, and congenital rubella. Associated problems are commonplace and include learning disability, cerebral palsy, hearing loss, language delay, and other congenital abnormalities.

Vision expidates the acquisition of skills such as exploring the environment, mobility, sound and touch location, and socialisation. Parents may socially interact less with visually impaired children due to a perceived lack of responsiveness. They need to learn to respond to vocalisation in active ways other than visual such as sound and touch. Object constancy is slower to develop and thus separation from an attachment figure, for example during hospitalisation, may be particularly traumatic. Other concepts difficult for the child to understand include continuity, time, and distance.

Moderate to severe psychiatric morbidity occurs in up to half of the visually impaired. The risk is increased in those with multiple disabilities, severe visual loss, psychiatric morbidity in the parents, the length of early hospitalisation, and the nature of family relationships. Stereotypies are common, particularly in those who are completely blind, and include hand flapping and rocking. These may result from understimulation or distress. Other problems characteristic of this group include social withdrawal, self-injurious behaviour, sleeping and feeding difficulties, and adjustment disorder.

Burns

Burns are the second most frequent cause of accidental death, after road traffic accidents, and about 15% of children hospitalised for burns are the result of child abuse such as immersion in hot fluid. The other at risk group comprises those involved in frequent accidents. This may be a result of the child's temperament or intracerebral pathology such as epilepsy, attention deficit hyperactivity disorder or subsequent to environmental factors such as overcrowding and deprived living conditions. The physical, emotional and interpersonal domains of the child's life may all be disturbed subsequent to the injury.

Physical aspects

Management requires controlling the severe pain, possible admission to an intensive care unit, and in some prolonged hospitalisation and rehabilitation. Repeated grafting, debridement and dressing changes may all be the precursors of further pain, anxiety and conflict between child, staff and parents. Both the staff and parents may experience guilt, the former as a consequence of having to perform painful dressing changes and the latter because they may feel that they could have prevented the injury and because of their inability to protect their child from pain. Scarring and contractures may result in marked changes in the child's physical appearance, with all the subsequent problems associated with disfigurement (see above).

Psychological aspects

Children may respond to the injury and its treatment with anything from opposition to regression, dependent clinging behaviour, and passive compliance. Sleep disturbance, poor self-esteem, post-traumatic stress disorder and depression may all develop subsequent to the burn. The child may develop a phobic avoidance of treatment that involves pain, with anxiety that may persist long after recovery from the burn.

Social aspects

The family may grieve the loss of their "perfect" child, develop depression or post-traumatic stress disorder. Some children, in addition to suffering from the burn, may be grieving the loss of a friend or relative subsequent to the same accident. In those where the injury is the result of abuse or pre-existing family psychopathology, a special assessment may be required.

Management

Management involves adequate analgesia, clear explanation of the treatment process and imparting the child with some sense of control over procedures. Antipsychotics for delirium and agitation, anxiolytics for anxiety and stress, and antidepressants are all useful when indicated.

Group and individual meetings with the family and child at all stages of recovery are therapeutic and particularly useful in discharge planning. Individual psychotherapy for the child should facilitate adjustment to the physical and emotional changes subsequent to the injury. The child may experience difficulty reintegrating into school and society, with increased sensitivity to teasing. A member of the team may prevent this with a school visit to help prepare teachers and children prior to the return of the child to school.

If the injury is the result of a suicidal attempt or other mental illness, this will require management in its own right.

Human immunodeficiency virus (HIV)

Children at risk of contracting HIV infection include those born to infected mothers (accounting for approximately 80% of paediatric HIV positive cases), recipients of contaminated blood transfusions, intravenous drug users, those sexually abused by HIV positive adults, the sexually promiscuous, and male homosexual adolescent boys.

The World Health Organisation estimates that HIV has infected approximately 1·5 million children since the pandemic began. The rates amongst the heterosexual population are increasing, with rates predicted to increase in those children born to HIV positive mothers. The highest rates worldwide are in Sub-Saharan Africa, South Asia and Urban India.

The child born to an HIV positive parent cannot be diagnosed as harbouring the infection until the maternal antibodies disappear. This occurs in the majority between 9 and 15 months of age. This time of uncertainty will be particularly stressful. The diagnosis in the child may be the time the mother learns that she is infected when she has thus far been asymptomatic. In some cases the mother may be too unwell to care for the child when substitute parenting may be necessary. Some children may have the added burden of losing their mother early on in life. Feelings of guilt can further complicate matters for parents.

Psychiatric manifestations of HIV infection

In up to 18% of cases progressive encephalopathy will be the presenting problem. It probably results from both direct and indirect effects of HIV infection on the brain. The neurological consequences include impaired brain growth, loss or plateauing of developmental milestones, progressive motor dysfunction, and other neurological signs. Approximately 18% of patients will have an abnormality on CT scan, such as cortical atrophy, ventricular dilatation, white matter abnormalities, and intracerebral calcification. Psychiatric and behavioural symptoms are common resulting from a number of factors such as CNS pathology, opportunistic infection, the chronic strain of the illness on the child and family, and malnutrition. Disorders that predominate include depression, attention deficit hyperactivity disorder, learning disorders, developmental delay, and anorexia nervosa.

Management

The management of these children requires a multidisciplinary approach, ideally in a specialist centre. Skills are required to identify developmental, neuropsychiatric and affective manifestations of the disease. Furthermore, support is required not only for the child but also the parents, who themselves may be HIV positive. All family members have to cope with the consequences of the infection, the fear of progression, concerns about infecting others, and the stigma.

All such children and families require a comprehensive package of health education, psychological and social support, family counselling, and individual therapies.

References

1 Graham P, Stevenson J, Flynn D. A new measure of health-related quality of life for children: preliminary findings. *Psychological Health* 1997;**12**:655–65.
2 Varni JW, Katz ER, Seid M, Quiggins DJ, Friedman-Bender A, Castro CM. The Pediatric Cancer Quality of Life Inventory (PCQL). 1. Instrument development, descriptive statistics, and cross-informant variance. *Journal of Behaviour Medicine* 1998;**21**:179–204.
3 Parkin PC, Kirpalani HM, Rosenbaum PL, *et al*. Development of a health-related quality of life instrument for use in children with spina bifida. *Quality of Life Research* 1997;**6**:123–132.
4 Juniper EF, Guyatt GH, Feeny DH, Griffith LE, Ferrie PJ. Minimum skills required by children to complete health related quality of life instruments for asthma: comparison of measurement properties. *European Respiratory Journal* 1997;**10**:2285–94.

5 Snyder CR, Hoza B, Pelham WE, *et al.* The development and validation of the Children's Hope Scale. *Journal of Pediatric Psychology* 1997;**22**:399–421.
6 Rauch PK, Jellinek MS, Murphy JM, *et al.* Screening for psychosocial dysfunction in a pediatric dermatology practice. *Clinical Pediatrics* 1991;**30**:8–14.

Further reading

Breslau N, Marshall IA. Psychological disturbance in children with physical disabilities: continuity and change in a five year follow up. *Journal of Abnormal Child Psychology* 1985;**13**:199–216.
Eiser C. Psychological effects of chronic disease. *Journal of Child Psychology and Psychiatry* 1990;**31**:85–98.
Freeman RD. Blind children's early emotional development: do we know enough to help? *Child: Care, Health and Development* 1989;**15**:3–28.
Fritz G. Factors in fatal childhood asthma. *American Journal of Orthopsychiatry* 1987;**57**:253–7.
Gillberg C. *Clinical child neuropsychiatry.* Cambridge: Cambridge University Press, 1995.
Golden MP, Ingersoll GM, Brack CJ, Russell BA, Wright JC, Huberty TJ. Longitudinal relationship of asymptomatic hypoglycaemia to cognitive function in IDDM. *Diabetes Care* 1989;**12**:89–93.
Gustafsson PA, Cederblad M, Ludvigsson J, *et al.* Family interaction and metabolic balance in juvenile diabetes mellitus. A prospective study. *Diabetes Research and Clinical Practice* 1987;**4**:7–14.
Knapp PK, Harris ES. Consultation—liaison in child psychiatry. A review of the past 10 years. Part 1. Clinical findings. *Journal of the American Academy of Child and Adolescent Psychiatry* 1998;**37**:17–25.
Lask B, Fosson A. *Childhood illness: the psychosomatic approach. Children talking with their bodies.* Wiley Series in Family Psychology. Chichester: John Wiley, 1989.
Meltzer H, Gatward R, Goodman R, Ford T. *The mental health of children and adolescence in Great Britain. A summary report*, 2nd edn. London: A National Statistics Publication, 2000.
Moores DF, Meadow-Orlans KP. *Educational and developmental aspects of deafness.* Washington, DC: Gallandet University Press, 1990.
Mrazek DA, Schuman WB, Klinnert M. Early asthma onset: risk of emotional and behavioural difficulties. *Journal of Child Psychology and Psychiatry* 1998;**39**:247–54.
Rotherum-Borus M. Children and HIV/AIDS. *Clinical Child Psychology and Psychiatry* 2002;**7**:7–124.

15: Psychological aspects of learning disability

Introduction

This chapter describes the psychological issues involved in caring for children with learning disability. The developmentally impaired carry a three to four times greater risk of developing a psychiatric illness than the general population. Indeed, 40% of those with learning disability have significant psychiatric symptomatology. Sadly, they are also at greater risk of exploitation and abuse.

Definition

Many terms have been used to describe this group, including mental handicap, mental retardation, developmental impairment, intellectual disability, learning disability, children with special needs. Different terms have probably been adopted in an attempt to dispel the prejudice which inevitably follows the label in vogue.

For the sake of convenience we shall use the one term "learning disability" defined as: "developmental intellectual impairment (IQ of 70 or less) with social disability".

Learning disability may be subdivided into:

- Mild (IQ of 50–70 or 2 SD below the mean)
- Moderate (IQ of 35–49)
- Severe (IQ of 20–34)
- Profound (IQ of below 20).

It is important to remember however that IQ should not be used in isolation to diagnose learning disability but in collaboration with functional ability. Indeed two children with the same IQ can vary considerably with regard to their skills, strengths, and temperaments. It is more helpful to think in terms of how these children's impairment leads to loss of function and thus social disadvantage.

Epidemiology

Learning disability affects approximately 1–3% of the population in the developed world. Mild learning disability is overrepresented amongst the lower socioeconomic groups especially with increasing numbers of siblings, overcrowded accommodation, and poverty. There has also been shown to be a significant contribution made by birth order, maternal ages at childbirth, and education level of the mother. Severe learning disability is influenced less by socioeconomic class and occurs at a rate between 0·3 and 0·5%.

Aetiology

Learning disability occurs in a number of disorders and comprises a variety of specific and non-specific pathological groups. With genetic advances, new genetically defined syndromes are being discovered regularly. Causes of increased psychopathology can be divided into biological, psychological, and sociocultural, though all three interact. In the severely impaired, biological factors (in approximately 55–75%) play a more prominant role. As would be expected, this group has larger associated medical complications, for example seizures increase with decreasing IQ. However in the mildly impaired, psychological and sociocultural factors are of greater importance.

Biological factors

In those with severe learning disability prenatal causes predominate, with other important causes including cerebral palsy, Down's syndrome, fragile X syndrome, chromosomal anomalies, single gene disorders, dysmorphic syndromes, idiopathic epilepsy, and fetal alcohol syndrome.

Perinatal and postnatal causes each account for a further 5% of the total. Only 10–25% of those with mild learning disability have resulted from an organic cause, those predominating including less severe cerebral palsy, idiopathic epilepsy, and dysmorphic syndromes.

Certain types of biological vulnerabilities predispose children with learning disability to specific psychopathology[1]:

- There is a higher incidence of autistic spectrum disorder in those with learning disability.
- Learning disability and epilepsy is particularly associated with psychosis and behavioural dyscontrol.
- Learning disability and motor impairments such as spina bifida and cerebral palsy are associated with hyperactivity and inattention.
- Learning disability and multiple sensory handicaps are particularly associated with emotional and behavioural problems.

Furthermore, those with learning disability may be prescribed medications for their epilepsy or disturbed behaviour, which may have psychiatric side effects.

Psychological factors

Children with reduced cognition have an impaired ability to solve problems and navigate their way through the demands of everyday life, resulting in anxiety, distress, and abnormal behaviour.

Psychological factors in the child

These children have less differentiated self-concepts. They may view themselves negatively, further exacerbated by failing tasks. They have a tendency to dependency, impulsivity, and social withdrawal.

Psychological factors in the family

Family coping depends on factors in the child such as IQ, age, and associated psychopathology, and factors in the family such as support, parental adjustment, marital harmony, and the perception of the child. The family may suffer unresolved grief resulting from the loss of a child for whom they had wished. This occasionally results in denial of the child's disability and "doctor shopping" for miracle cures. There may be an overinvolved and enmeshed relationship between mother and child excluding other members of the family, with infantilisation of the child. There may be feelings of guilt associated with self-blaming and impaired limit setting of the child's behaviour. However, most parents make the adjustment slowly but surely, coming to appreciate their children for who and what they are, rather than what they might have been. For many parents positives are found that many clinicians overlook or dismiss too readily.

Those with a learning disability are at particular risk of maltreatment, be it physical or sexual abuse or exploitation. They also suffer social stigma affecting their opportunities of socialisation and employment, reducing self-esteem with resultant feelings of isolation. Those with learning disability may be more dependent on others and thus more vulnerable to the effects of loss of a carer with resultant disturbed behaviour.

Features of psychopathology

The clinical picture can vary greatly depending on the underlying aetiology of the learning disability. Personality factors, associated disorders (for example epilepsy) and psychosocial differences account for further variation within syndromes.

Those with mild learning disability display the full plethora of psychopathology seen in the "normal" population. The moderate and severe learning disability groups also experience the same psychiatric disorders as the normal population but with modified symptoms. In addition, they suffer symptoms which can not readily be classified as a standard psychiatric disorder, and one is therefore left exploring the factors contributing to the symptom and its meaning.

Those with profound learning disability usually have insufficient motor or expressive behaviour for the emergence of psychopathology.

Psychopathology is particularly problematic in the severely and moderately impaired because their degree of disability results in:

- Suffering to the individual through self-injury and trauma to vital sensory organs such as ears and eyes.
- Family distress.
- Distress in residential staff, who are caring for those with higher levels of psychiatric disturbance than their community counterparts.
- Behavioural disturbance which interferes with possibilities for independent living.
- Financial burden on the family, agencies, and the community.

Two mistakes are often made with these children:

1. Their behavioural symptoms are rationalised as being part of their learning disability and a superimposed psychiatric disorder is overlooked.
2. They are overmedicated with neuroleptics for inadequate or ill-defined reasons, with resultant serious side effects (to which they are particularly prone).

It is sometimes a challenge to discern whether behaviour is an expression of emotional distress or a manifestation of the learning disability. Consideration should be given to how the patient's behaviour relates to developmental age, taking into account the verbal limitation of the child in describing inner feelings, and utilising parental and carer reports as well as any other sources of information. Using experience gained from working with young children can help in relating to those with similar developmental age.

A brief summary of the clinical features of those with learning disability is provided, followed by the associated disabilities and features of psychiatric disorders. Specific behavioural patterns associated with different syndromes are outlined in Table 15.1.

Mild learning disability (IQ 50–70)

Approximately 80% of those with learning disability are in this category. Such children tend to be of normal appearance with minimal motor deficits, and normal language and social skills. As adults they will often live independently, though many require assistance with housing, employment, and

Table 15.1 Specific learning disability syndromes and behavioural phenotypes

Syndrome	Pathophysiology	Average level of disability (LD)	Behavioural and psychological characteristics	Physical phenotype
Fragile X Prevalence 0·5 – 1 per 1000. Accounts for approximately 10% of mental retardation in males	Inactivation of FMR – 1 gene at Xq 27·3 due to CGG base repeats with high gene methylation plus subsequent reduced FMRIP (fragile X protein). Fully affected male = NO FMRIP. Displays dynamic mutation	Males: moderate LD, one third profound LD Females: normal to mild LD. Cognitive deficits include short term memory deficit, visual-motor coordination, mathematics and attention deficits Relative strengths: verbal long term memory	Commonest inherited cause of LD. Spectrum of difficulties in relating to others. Males: more severe with autism in 15–25%, others show social anxiety, withdrawal, gaze aversion, slow-to-warm-up shyness. Most understand emotions in others. ADHD common Females: depression, reduced interpersonal skills, anxious perseveration	Males: long narrow face, large prominent ears, macrocephaly, prominent jaw and forehead, joint hypermobility, postpubertal macro–orchidism, mitral valve prolapse, protruding lower lip Females: features less marked but similar in type In both genders features more prominent post puberty
Down's syndrome Prevalence approximately 1% per 1000 live births related to maternal age: 0·5 : 1000 women age 20 years;	95% have full trisomy 21 (not inherited), 5% translocation usually between chromosomes 14 and 21 (may be inherited), 1% mosaics	Mild to profound learning disability. Speech and language delay	Commonest genetic cause of severe learning disability. The stereotype of being happy, good tempered and placid has not been validated. No one	Reduced stature, growth retardation in limbs more than trunk. Facial features — marked brachycephaly with decreased anteroposterior diameter, flattened face

(Continued)

Table 15.1 (*Continued*)

Syndrome	Pathophysiology	Average level of disability (LD)	Behavioural and psychological characteristics	Physical phenotype
1 : 1000 women age 30 years. Approximately 10% women age 49 years			particular behavioural phenotype. Delayed walking usually after 2 years. Less psychopathology than in other developmentally delayed group, though more than in the general population. Most psychiatric disorders seen and include, in particular, attentional deficits, impulsivity, aggression, and hyperactivity. Autistic spectrum disorder relatively rare. At risk for Alzheimer's dementia generally presenting clinically after 50 years	with outward and upward slant of the eyes and epicanthal folds, low nasal root and small nose, low-set dysplastic ears, white spots in central part of iris (Brushfield spots) and increased incidence of cataracts and squints. The mouth is small and tongue appears large and fissured. Hands are short, little finger is inward curving (clinodactyly), and there is a single palmar (simian) crease. The foot shows wide space between big and second toes. There is hypotonia and hypermobility of joints and often cardiac atrioventricular septal defect and duodenal stenosis. There is an increased prevalence of autoimmune

(Continued)

Table 15.1 (Continued)

Syndrome	Pathophysiology	Average level of disability (LD)	Behavioural and psychological characteristics	Physical phenotype
				problems including leukaemia as well as thyroid dysfunction, for example hypothyroidism. Hearing defects are common, particularly of the conductive type
Prader-Willi syndrome Prevalence 1 : 10–20 000 live births	Between 60% and 80% microdeletion on chromosome 15, paternal origin at the locus 15q 11–13. Most of the remainder have two copies of the maternal chromosome and no paternal contribution—uniparental disomy	Mild to moderate LD. 50% of individuals with IQ greater than 70. Strengths in puzzle solving and visual organisation and expressive vocabulary	Good natured with outbursts of rage. Emotional lability, skin picking, and scratching. Daytime hypersomnia. Anxiety and obsessive compulsive symptoms significantly increased	Infantile hypotonia and failure to thrive, subsequent hyperphagia, obesity and hoarding. 20% have reduced glucose tolerance. Small hands and feet, micro-orchidism, cryptorchidism, and micropenis. Almond shaped eyes, fair hair, light skin, flat face and prominent forehead with short stature.
Angelman's syndrome Prevalence very rare, around 1 : 30 000 live births	Deletion or rearrangement of the long arm of	Severe LD, absence of speech	Poor social skills, attentional deficits with hyperactivity. Feeding	Seizures, jerky, unsteady wide based gait, with hand flapping, outbursts of

(Continued)

Table 15.1 (Continued)

Syndrome	Pathophysiology	Average level of disability (LD)	Behavioural and psychological characteristics	Physical phenotype
	chromosome 15q11–13 in maternally derived chromosome. Very rarely uniparental disomy—paternal		problems in infancy, delayed ambulation and pica have been reported. Reduced need for sleep has been seen with happy disposition— "Happy Puppet"	laughter, and hydrophilia. Facial characteristics include: prominent chin, fair hair, microcephaly, maxillary hypoplasia and large mouth, blue eyes common. Characteristic EEG
Lesch–Nyhan syndrome Prevalence 1 : 10 000 to 1 : 38 000 live births	Congenital deficiency of purine salvage enzyme hypoxanthine guanine phosphoribosyltransferase resulting from mutation in the corresponding gene on the long arm of the x chromosome Xq 26–27, recessive	Moderate to severe LD	Self-mutilation is severe and includes biting of lips, fingers. Aggressive behaviour, anxiety and coprolalia in some	In males results in hyperuricaemia, spasticity, choreoathetosis, seizures, kidney failure, gout, and renal calculi. Heterozygous carrier females are generally clinically normal
Smith–Magenis syndrome Prevalence 1 : 500 000	Microdeletion on short arm of chromosome 17p11-2	Intellectual impairment is variable	Autistic features, hyperactivity (in 75%), inattention, self-injury such as head banging, nail pulling, and hand	Bradydactyly, broad face, flat midface and hoarse voice, though features subtle making diagnosis difficult

(Continued)

Table 15.1 (Continued)

Syndrome	Pathophysiology	Average level of disability (LD)	Behavioural and psychological characteristics	Physical phenotype
			biting. Nocturnal and diurnal enuresis. Sleep disorders with initial and middle insomnia and reduced or absent REM	
Williams syndrome Prevalence 1 : 20 000 live births	Associated with deletion in elastin gene at 7q11–23	Low average to mild LD. Weakness in visual spatial skills and visuomotor integration. Communication style loquacious, pseudo-mature, known as "cocktail party speech", present in approximately 40%	Tendency toward being socially outgoing — disinhibited. Hyperactive, anxious and stubborn, poor peer relationships, sleep and eating disturbances and hyperacusis is common	Facial characteristics: elfin faces, medial eyebrow flare, hypertelorism, stellate pattern of iris, periorbital fullness, drooping cheeks, long philtrum and fish lips. Large open mouth, upturned nose, low-set ears and short stature. Cardiac abnormalities include supravalvular aortic stenosis, peripheral pulmonary stenosis, and coarctation of the aorta. Hypercalcaemia is an important neonatal association as well as thyroid disorders

(Continued)

Table 15.1 (Continued)

Syndrome	Pathophysiology	Average level of disability (LD)	Behavioural and psychological characteristics	Physical phenotype
Cri du chat Prevalence 1 : 50 000 live births	Sporadic terminal deletion of chromosome 5p	Profound LD with limited speech	Infant has characteristic cry likened to kitten. Hyperactive, self stimulating behaviour, irritable and destructive	Microephaly, micrognathia, growth failure. Faces tend to be round and flat with hypetelorism, epicanthal folds, with antimongoloid slant to palpebral fissures, broad flat nose and low-set ears. Congenital heart disease and gastrointes-tinal abnormalities.
Cornelia de lange syndrome Prevalence at least 1 : 50 000 live births	Unknown, some have reported abnormalities of chromosome 3	Severe to profound LD. In the severe, limited speech and language delay	Severe self-injury, social withdrawal, autistic spectrum disorder	Short stature, short neck, small hands and feet. Contracted elbows, generalised hirsutism with synophrys, hairy ears, and micrognathia. Microcephaly, ante-verted nose, prominent philtrum and short upper lip. Shortened radius and finger hypoplasia common

(Continued)

Table 15.1 (Continued)

Syndrome	Pathophysiology	Average level of disability (LD)	Behavioural and psychological characteristics	Physical phenotype
Rubinstein – Taybi syndrome Prevalence 1 : 250 000 approximately	Most cases sporadic, in some documented microdeletion 16p 13·3	Expressive language difficulties—performance IQ > verbal IQ	Sociable, distractable, reduced concentration, mood lability, temper tantrums and self-stimulating behaviour	Microcephaly, ptosis, antimongoloid slant to eyes, strabismus, hooked nose, broad nasal bridge with nasal septum extending below alae. Broad thumb and toes, generalised hirsutism and short stature. Congenital heart disease, seizures (25%), EEG abnormalities in 75%
Tuberous sclerosis Prevalence 1 : 10 000 live births	Autosomal dominant. Abnormal proliferation of nerve cells resulting in benign (hamartomas) and more rarely malignant brain tumours	LD in 70%	Hyperactivity, autistic spectrum disorder in up to 80%. Self-injurious behaviours and sleep disturbances including middle and terminal insomnia	Butterfly-shaped skin lesion (adenoma sebaceum) over nasal bridge and cheek. Skin fibroma (shagreen patch) classically in the lumbosacral area, retinal phakoma and areas of skin depigmentation often oval shape. Associated multiple tumours in kidney, spleen, heart, and lungs. Epilepsy

(Continued)

Table 15.1 (Continued)

Syndrome	Pathophysiology	Average level of disability (LD)	Behavioural and psychological characteristics	Physical phenotype
				(infantile spasms, partial or generalised seizures).
Neurofibromatosis type 1. Prevalence 1 : 3 500	Autosomal dominant. Neurocutaenous condition. NFI allele mutated; NFI gene 17q 11:2	10% moderate to profound LD. Verbal IQ> performance IQ	Anxious distractible impulsive and hyperkinetic. Autism has been described in some	Multiple café-au-lait spots, axillary freckling developing usually during adolescence, neurofibromas, optic glioma, iris hamartomas, osseous lesion. Short stature and macrocephaly in approximately 35%. Epilepsy
Fetal alcohol syndrome Prevalence 1 : 600 to 1 : 3 000	Maternal alcohol consumption particularly in second and third trimester	Mild to moderate LD, speech and language deficits	Inattentive, reduced abstraction, impulsive, irritable and increased rates of depression	Prenatal and postnatal growth retardation, microcephaly, midfacial, hypoplasia, microphthalmia, thin upper lip with poorly defined philtrum and short stature. Cardiac anomalies
Klinefelter's syndrome Prevalence 1 : 500 newborn males	XXY — extra X chromosome consequent to abnormal separation in oogenesis or spermatogenesis	IQ usually in normal range with less than 20% having IQ below 90. Speech and language impairment	Anxious, dependent, socially withdrawn and increased rates of emotional disorder	Increased stature with obesity, gynaecomastia, delayed puberty with underdeveloped sexual characteristics and infertility

interpersonal responsibilities. They have a normal life expectancy. Other family members may well have a lowered IQ and belong to a lower socioeconomic group. Neglect is more common than in the other groups. One of the biggest difficulties is the failure of others to recognise their disability and the lack of services for them.

In the mildly intellectually impaired the association with physical disability is high but to a lesser degree than in the severe (see below) and profound groups.

Moderate learning disability (IQ 35–49)

Approximately 12% have moderate learning disability. Most are able to learn communication skills and to care for themselves with supervision, but few lead an independent life.

Severe learning disability (IQ 20–34)

Severe learning disability accounts for 7% of this group. They invariably have marked impairment in social functioning, require close supervision with self-care, and with time may learn to communicate in a simple way, for example using a signing system such as Makaton. They require clear structure in their daily lives. Physically they often display dysmorphic features, have motor deficits, major health problems such as epilepsy, and have shortened life expectancy with lowered fertility. The types of central nervous pathology associated with severe learning disability are cerebral palsy (21%), epilepsy (37%), visual (15%) and hearing impairment (8%), hydrocephalus (5%), and autism (8%).[2]

The rest of the family will usually be of normal IQ and neglect is unusual.

Profound learning disability (IQ below 20)

This group accounts for less than 1% of the total. They cannot care for themselves and social and language skills are at best elementary. They require full time care.

Specific psychiatric illness comorbid with learning disability

Mental illnesses frequently exist comorbidly with learning disabilities, with prevalence rates ranging from 30% to 70%. However, underdiagnosis is common due to the assumption that symptoms are manifestations of learning disability, non-specific and atypical clinical presentations, or as a result of "diagnostic overshadowing", i.e. when disruptive behaviours distract the clinician from a more global evaluation of the patient.

Practically all categories of mental illness are represented in this population. Some common comorbid mental disorders are considered below. The frequency of problems varies with age, with common reasons for referral in the very young being based around eating and sleep disorders. In the school age group attention deficit hyperactivity disorder (ADHD) and aggression become more frequent. Adolescent issues cluster around socialisation, sexuality, mood, and self-injury.

Attention deficit hyperactivity disorder

ADHD (see chapter 5) is a common presenting problem in those with learning disability, occurring at rates higher than in the general population. If chronological age alone is considered ignoring their developmental age, then they almost all will have deficits in attention. The diagnosis can be made using observable behaviour in a number of different situations, reported by multiple informants. Care needs to be taken not to confuse situation specific inattentiveness (for example at school resulting from overambitious academic expectations), medication side effects, or syndrome related behaviours. As with all aspects of assessing these children, the single most helpful perspective is to consider their behaviour within a developmental frame.

Disruptive disorders

Approximately 33% of those with mild learning disability will have an associated disruptive disorder (see chapter 5). When making a diagnosis consider the individual's circumstances and ability to comprehend social rules, as well as the acquisition of sufficient skills to be deliberately oppositional.

Mood disorders

Depressed mood (see chapter 6) occurs more frequently in those with learning disabilities than in the general population. In those with mild learning disability presentations are similar to those with normal intelligence, though complaints may be more concrete. Emphasis should be placed on observer ratings of mood changes from baseline or aggressive behaviour, which may mask a depressive aetiology. A search needs to be made for environmental triggers.

Mania also occurs with overactivity, excitement, irritability, nervousness, and sleep reduction. However it will need to be distinguished from other causes of hyperactivity.

Schizophrenia and psychotic disorders

The prevalence of schizophrenia in those with learning disabilities is similar to that in those without. It generally does not occur until late adolescence. It is characterized by disorganised behaviour, poverty of thought, catatonia, elaborate delusions, simple and repetitive hallucinations, with worsening social and intellectual functioning (see chapter 12). An organic cause needs to be excluded and care must be taken not to misinterpret conversations with imaginary friends as hallucinations. Striking out or shouting at empty space are clues to the presence of hallucinations.

Anxiety disorders

Anxiety disorder occurs in about 25% of those with learning disabilities. Psychosocial factors such as reduced self-esteem, fear of failing and loss of caregivers may contribute. Patients may prefer to talk about dislike of certain situations as opposed to fear. In those with poor verbal ability, reliance on observation of avoidance behaviours such as school refusal and visible signs of autonomic arousal are necessary. This group is also at an increased risk of suffering from post-traumatic stress disorder (see chapter 4) subsequent to their increased vulnerability to abuse and difficulties in subsequently reporting it.

Obsessive compulsive disorder (OCD)

Repetitive behaviours such as washing, tidying and arranging, which appear compulsive or driven and unwelcome, may indicate OCD spectrum behaviour. Care needs to be taken in differentiating this behaviour from the repetitive desire for sameness behaviour in the autistic spectrum disorder and self-stimulating stereotypies.

Stereotypic and self-injurious behaviour

Stereotypies are repetitive, non-goal-directed movements. They include head banging, rocking, hair pulling, nail biting, hand wringing, biting of limbs, and eyepoking. When they result in body damage it is described as self-injurious behaviour. This behaviour occurs particularly in those with severe learning disabilities and in those with autism.

This stereotypic and self-injurious behaviour can be understood as a mode of communication in those with few options to express needs. Not surprisingly the frequency of this behaviour increases in those with restricted mobility, sensory deficits (for example impaired vision), and communication difficulties. The context of the behaviour can be in both an understimulating or overstimulating and demanding environment.

Disorders that are particularly associated with such behaviour include, Rett's, Lesch–Nyhan, Cornelia de lange, Prader–Willi, Smith-Magenis and fragile X syndromes.

Eating difficulties

Although anorexia nervosa and bulimia nervosa (see chapter 8) are very rare in those with learning disabilities, both overeating and undereating may occur. Overeating is often a response to boredom and undereating to depression. Failure to thrive, pica and rumination with regurgitation and chewing of food are common.

Autistic spectrum disorder (ASD)

In those with a diagnosis of ASD, two thirds will have an IQ less than 70. Likewise 1% of those with learning disabilities will have ASD. However autistic-like syndromes that do not fulfil the criteria of ASD are far more common in those with severe LD (see chapter 16).

Mental illness arising from a missed medical disorder

Care needs to be taken to exclude the possibility that the psychiatric illness is not secondary to the consequences of medical conditions or personality changes subsequent to the emergence of seizures. Medical possibilities include pain that the patient is unable to communicate, dental caries, covert infection (for example, tonsillitis), anaemia, malnutrition, space occupying lesions, foreign bodies, degenerative disease, endocrine problems, accidental poisoning, epilepsy, drug side effects, and congenital abnormal neuroanatomy and function.

Assessment

The principles of a psychiatric assessment remain the same in learning disabilities as for non-cognitively impaired individuals (see chapter 2). In those with impaired communication skills, more emphasis needs to be placed on the caregivers' observations.

Issues to be considered include:

- All aspects of functioning including deficits and strengths, ability to self-care, interpersonal functioning, academic skills, play, and health risk issues.
- The function of the behaviour—what is the child trying to communicate?
- Is the behaviour situation specific?
- Analyse the symptoms in terms of:

  - *Antecedents*—what precedes it?
  - *Behaviour*—the precise description of the behaviour
  - *Consequences*—what management measures are used and what are the results? Is bad behaviour inadvertently being reinforced?

- Review past cognitive tests, including subtest scores, noting areas of strength and weakness, and consider the need for further evaluation.

- Compare current with past behaviour, personality, and mood.
- Explore any past psychiatric illnesses, response and side effects to medication, psychotherapies, and behavioural treatments.
- Delineate all sources of support, and stress any recent changes or losses in caregivers, family and teachers, and always consider the possibility of physical and sexual abuse.
- Establish what is the parents'/caregivers' understanding of the problem and disability, their attitude towards the child, and whether growth is nurtured or the child is overprotected or rejected.

In the interview, which may best be conducted at home or the school, allow sufficient time, ensure questions are understood, using clear and concrete language. If the use of interpreters is necessary, such as in those with hearing deficits, still direct the questions at the patient. One should move from talking about the patient's strengths via neutral material to the problem at hand. Care should be taken to avoid closed, overly specific questions to start with. Non-verbal techniques include observation of performance at various tasks such as attention span, activity level, emotional expression, play, and artwork.

A thorough medical review and examination excludes medical causes of behavioural symptoms. The assessment should explore the patients' strengths, deficits, needs, adaptive behaviour, communication, health, and psychosocial domains. This can be assisted by using the multiaxial classification suggested by the Royal College of Psychiatrists (Box 15.1).[3]

Treatment

As with patients without learning disabilities, optimal care will include a multifaceted multidisciplinary approach, using similar principles. The main tenets of care include parental counselling (see chapter 22), behavioural approaches (see chapter 24), family therapy (see chapter 22), and psychopharmacology (see chapter 25). In all cases family issues need to be considered.

> **Box 15.1 The Royal College of Psychiatrists multiaxial classification**
> 1. Life context — home, family, occupation where appropirate
> 2. Cognitive level and mental age — IQ if available; specify test used and date
> 3. Development disorders, for example speech and language deficits
> 4. Organic factos — include aetiology of handicap, such as genetic syndrome and any concurrent illness
> 5. Psychosocial factors including quality of friendships and relationships
> 6. Psychiatric and behavioural state — include understanding of handicap, insight, and self-esteem
> 7. Functional abilities such as self-care and communication

Parental counselling and family therapy

Parental counselling includes educating the parents about their child's condition, giving advice about management, educational facilities and local support groups, and helping parents to find their own solutions.

At the time of diagnosis parents may react with grief, anger, and despair. They will need help in recognising their child's strengths, and in dealing with their feelings of guilt and desire to overprotect. Behavioural management plans derived at school will need to be generalised to the home, so close links should be fostered between parents, teachers and other service providers such as speech therapists. The parents may need support at critical times such as puberty, transition to secondary school, or entering residential care.

Behavioural therapy

The goal is to promote realistically achievable desirable behaviour, as well as to extinguish undesirable behaviour (in some, complete abolition of unwanted behaviour may not be realistic). Behaviour therapy (see chapter 24) can be used across all levels of learning disabilities, being particularly useful in the severe range, and can be targeted to manage aggression, self-injury, toilet training and to promote self-help skills.

In severe situations where the behaviour is harmful such as self-injury, quick results may be necessary. These can be achieved by using such techniques as time out, i.e. removing the child from a rewarding environment to a quiet non-stimulating room for very short periods of time. Alternatively, a harshly spoken "No" may act as a simple aversive intervention in some children. Protective clothing such as gloves for self-injurious behaviour may be required.

Individual psychotherapy

This population group can benefit from individual psychotherapy providing that approaches are adapted to their needs and basic communication skills are present.

The therapy needs to be modified to the developmental stage and communication skills of the patient. Whether cognitive behavioural therapy or psychodynamic approaches are used, the therapist needs to be active, directive, flexible, and supportive, and be able to give concrete advice. Concrete goals should be set with the aim to achieve the best quality of life. Areas that may be focused on include self-image, understanding their disability, developing strengths and talents, independence, and social skills where appropriate.

Group therapy

Group therapy is particularly beneficial in adolescents with relatively good verbal skills. It is a good arena for providing support, education, interpretation, and cooperation. Role playing can be used in developing social skills.

Pharmacotherapy

Pharmacotherapy should be considered in the context of a comprehensive treatment approach, and preferably with advice from those experienced in prescribing in this group. For the specifics of medication used see chapter 25. Where appropriate baseline electrocardiogram and blood tests should be performed. Compared with the non-intellectually impaired community there is less information about the safety and efficacy of psychotropic medication, particularly in children. Most medication is not specifically licensed in this group and support for its use is based on extrapolation of the effects in adults or normal children. It therefore may be appropriate, where consent is tenuous or fluctuating, to elicit written consent, having explained that the use of medication lies outside of approved criteria, even though clinical literature upholds its use.

General principles include: treating each case as a single case study, starting with commonly used drugs, with the safest profile, at the lowest dose, increasing in small increments. Review the need for medication regularly. This group is particularly sensitive to anticholinergic side effects, extrapyramidal side effects, the disinhibiting effects of sedative-hypnotic agents, and the neuroleptic malignant syndrome. Therefore warn the carer of side effects, especially the common and serious ones. When selecting a drug, consider which medication is most likely to ameliorate the target symptom and other behavioural disturbances present.

Challenging behaviour

When aggression arises from a psychiatric disorder, for example ADHD, bipolar disorder, then the treatment for the disorder will provide the best response. Where aggression arises from fear, mood instability, or impulsivity, the underlying emotion should be targeted. However, there are only a few studies showing the efficacy of antipsychotics in the absence of psychosis.

Haloperidol or diazepam can be helpful. Future trials may endorse the use of newer atypical antipsychotics for this purpose. Clinical studies have shown some benefits with serotonergic agents such as buspirone, which decreases anxiety and may help self-injurious behaviour and aggression.

Before choosing any drugs explain simply the potential therapeutic benefits and side effects. This has to be pitched at the intellectual level of the child where possible. The least detrimental option should be chosen, weighing up benefit against side effects and considering the child's quality of life. Informed consent may not be possible in this group, in which case the parent or caregiver with parental responsibility needs to be even more actively involved in the decision making process.

Conclusion

Although there are surprisingly few studies of intervention for children with psychiatric disorders comorbid with learning disabilities these children and their families do seem to benefit from treatment. Indications for use of medication for challenging behaviour needs further clarification but there is now a much more optimistic view on the role of medication in the armamentarium of care. Different treatment options need to be made available and accessible through the development of appropriate services to help children, adolescents and their families to lead an improved quality of life. It is often a surprise to less seasoned practitioners that these patients and their families can be amongst the most satisfying to treat.

References

1 Dykens EM. Annotation: psychopathology in children with intellectual disability. *Journal of Child Psychology and Psychiatry* 2000;**41**:407–17.
2 Gillberg C, ed. Mental retardation and other severe learning disabilities. An overview. In: *Clinical child neuropsychiatry*. Cambridge: Cambridge University Press, 1995:45–53.
3 Anness V. A multi-aspect assessment for people with mental handicap. *Psychiatric Bulletin* 1991;**15**:146.

Further reading

Bernet W, Dulcan M. Practice parameters for the assessment and treatment of children, adolescents and adults with mental retardation and comorbid mental disorders. (Practice Parameters: AACAP Official Action.) *Journal of the American Academy of Child and Adolescent Psychiatry* 1999;**38**:5S–31S.
Dossetor D. The hit and miss of magic bullets: a guide to psychotropic medication for young people with intellectual handicap. *Clinical Child Psychology and Psychiatry* 1997;**2**:65–93.
King BH, State MW. Mental retardation. In: Klykylo WM, Kay J, Rube D, eds. *Clinical child psychiatry*. Philadelphia: WB Saunders, 1998:356–80.
Minnes P. Mental retardation: the impact upon the family. In: Bunck JA, Hodapp RM, Zigler E, eds. *Handbook of mental retardation and development*. New York: Cambridge University Press, 1998:693–712.
Santosh PJ, Baird G. Psychopharmacotherapy in children and adults with intellectual disability (seminar). *Lancet* 1999;**354**(9174):233–42.

16: Autistic spectrum disorders

Introduction

Autistic spectrum disorders are a group of syndromes that include autism, Asperger's syndrome, and Rett's syndrome. The core features of this group of disorders are impaired social interaction and communication, stereotypic behaviours or obsessional interests and activities, and cognitive impairment.

Autism

Autism is manifested by an onset, by the age of 3 years, of disturbance of reciprocal social interaction, communication abnormalities and restricted, stereotyped and repetitive patterns of behaviour and interests.

Epidemiology

Autism affects approximately 0·5–1 in 1000 children with a male to female ratio of 3 to 1.

Clinical picture

Abnormal development is apparent before the age of 3 years with a constellation of disturbances in social interaction and communication, and restricted and repetitive interests and behaviour.

Disturbed social interaction

There is an inability to form relationships with age peers, and poorly developed empathy skills (the ability to understand how others feel and think). Imitation play is lacking and typically eye contact is avoided. Additionally the quality of gaze is different, being more fixed ("stiffer") and longer lasting than in non-autistic individuals. Many resist being touched or held, though they can enjoy body contact if they initiate it. The difficulty these children have in interacting often makes it hard for others to warm to them. Parents may feel guilty about their own lack of engendered warmth.

Abnormalities of communication development

From an early age there are problems comprehending gesture and speech, with a definite delay in the development and comprehension of spoken language. One in two children with autism fails to develop useful spoken language, and in those who do it is abnormal in form. The communication lacks a social to and fro, often being repetitious or taking on the form of a monologue. As a result of their inability to communicate with the "inner worlds" of others, they learn through copying what they see and hear. They may refer to themselves as "you" or "he", repeat words in a meaningless way (echolalia), or take on stereotypical speech heard in others and used in the wrong context. Abnormalities in intonation, rhythm and pitch may also be present (dysprosidy).

Comprehension of spoken language is compromised. Though many understand individual words, problems arise when these are sequenced together. There is no understanding of metaphor, irony, sarcasm, and exaggeration, however the use of adult speech and the absence of expression of feelings may give a pseudomature or even pseudoprofound quality to the speech.

Non-verbal communication problems include poor judgement of interpersonal distance, prolonged eye gaze, eye closure, or inappropriate looking at mouths rather than eyes. There may be anything from restricted to absent bodily and facial gestures. Object sharing and pointing is notably limited.

Parents and teachers may experience the communication difficulties as an inability to "get through to them" or an experience of being "locked out".

Restricted and repetitive interests and behaviour

Autistic children display stereotypical behaviours and interests. They may become preoccupied by a specific part of a toy, or interested in the particular sensory property of an object such as its taste, texture, colour, or smell. Toys may be lined up for hours on end. Attachments may form to unusual objects such as locks of hair or bottle caps.

Play is typically neither symbolic nor imaginative with rigid and restrictive play patterns and interests. The child may have a very restricted diet and from time to time stop eating completely for no apparent reason. Certain routines are adhered to in a rigid way with minor changes causing extreme reactions. Conversely, major life events may not be registered.

During the school years preoccupations or special interests such as maps, weather reports and train schedules may develop. Simple stereotypies such as hand flapping, tiptoe walking, finger twirling, spinning and rocking are often exhibited. Parents are often confused as to whether they should accommodate to these behaviours or attempt to modify them.

Abnormal responses to sensory stimuli

From a very young age abnormal responses to sensory stimuli may be present, sometimes misleading the clinician into suspecting that the child is either blind or deaf. Extreme responses and sensitivity to sound may be seen, such as ignoring explosions to covering ears when the wrapper of a sweet is removed.

Though light touch or stroke may result in withdrawal, children may deliberately bite and burn body parts or bang their head. If the feel of faeces is particularly of interest to the child, faecal smearing may be prominent or even tension relieving.

Responses to visual stimuli may include a fascination with contrasts of light and peering at objects in unusual ways and with peripheral vision.

Concomitant hyperactivity and food fads are common.

The striking feature is the loss of commensurability of response to stimulus—a loss of "fine tuning".

Intelligence

About three quarters of autistic individuals have an IQ below 70, with IQ being the most powerful predictor of outcome. Regardless of IQ there is a distinctive cognitive profile with strong visuospatial skills and poor symbolisation, understanding of abstract ideas and creative skills. A minority show islets of special abilities ("autistic savant"), such as numerical skills, calendar skills and in the field of music and art.

Associated disabilities

There are a number of associated difficulties including hearing impairment in approximately 20%, visual problems such as refractive errors and squints, expressive dysphasia superimposed on language abnormalities in about 20% and epilepsy developing in 25% by adolescence.

Associated medical conditions

Conditions associated with autism at a rate higher than in the general population include:

- Fragile X syndrome
- Tuberous sclerosis
- Neurofibromatosis
- Rett's syndrome
- Hypomelanosis of Ito
- Moebius syndrome
- Rubella.

Aetiology

At present the precise cause of autism is unknown, however it seems that at least in some cases genetic factors are involved. Studies of twins reveal over 90% concordance for autism in monozygotic twins compared to 0% in dizygotic twins. Rutter has proposed that the disorder results from an inherited cognitive deficit coupled with an environmental insult. The current debate about the role of the triple vaccine (MMR) remains unresolved. The orthodox medical establishment is strongly dismissive of the suggestion, but there is a vocal minority who are more open-minded.

Assessment

A full physical examination should be performed particularly looking for any associated medical conditions.

A neurodevelopmental examination should be performed and the child's cognitive level and language abilities determined.

Investigations

The following investigations are recommended to exclude various medical conditions:

- Chromosomal analysis looking for fragile X, XYY, deletions and partial tetrasomy 15
- CT/MRI scan
- EEG
- Audiological testing—hearing test, auditory brainstem response examination
- Ophthalmology assessment
- Speech assessment
- Metabolic screen of urine.

Management

Rutter has described four basic aims in treating an autistic individual:[1]

1. Foster social and communicative development.
2. Enhance learning and problem solving without overtaxing the child.
3. Decrease behaviours that interfere with learning and access to opportunities for normal experience.
4. Help families cope.

Counselling and behavioural approaches are the cornerstone of treatment. Intensive psychotherapeutic approaches rarely if ever benefit.

Education

Diagnostic information It is important to give a clear diagnosis with information about the condition and investigations to parents, relatives, and other carers. Seminars and self-help groups are helpful. Parents often find attempts to make "contact" frustrating and in the end deeply saddening. It may be helpful to point out that this is much more painful for them than for the child.

The impact upon siblings is often considerable and their needs are often inadvertently overlooked.

A structured environment A high level of predictability needs to be created incorporating routines acceptable to child and adult alike. Education of the child needs structure and consistency in terms of time, room, and teacher. Instructions should be given one at a time, allowing time to finish one task before proceeding to the next.

There is a fine line between overstimulation and understimulation. Too little to do and lack of structure may have a similar impact as too much to do and too much structure.

Behavioural programme Autistic children do not learn automatically from new experiences and interactions. All learning needs have to be gained through training. Individual skills and deficits are identified and then training-needs planned. When an integrated educational/behavioural modification programme is organised, it should be created in collaboration with parents. In general, learning takes place through procedures rather than words.

Making sure treatments generalise to daily care It is important to individualise the child's treatment to the child's own personality, IQ, and social background. Approaches to autism based in the home benefit the child and family more directly than clinic-based programmes. Concentration should be on daily life activities such as feeding, hygiene, toileting, dressing, hair care, and sleeping. Spoken language should be simplified as much as possible because of the problems of understanding.

Teaching communication skills

A combination of non-verbal methods of communication, such as sign language and symbols, as well as verbal methods may result in better communication than either alone. Using pictures and symbols or photographs as aids in communicating may be helpful.

Speech therapy will help the child take part in structured conversations, increasing spontaneous communication and enlarging vocabulary. Help can be given in obtaining appropriate eye contact, turn taking, and how to hold conversations.

The child must learn by rote what is unconsciously acquired and "obvious" in normal children.

Schooling

The aim is to find the least restrictive educational environment for the particular child, depending on individual needs. This may mean for some a classroom specifically designed for autistic children. Alternatively a classroom for the child with a communication handicap may be more appropriate. Others may find a classroom for the developmentally delayed the most comfortable environment. Finally a few may be best integrated into a normal school.

Usually schooling is a compromise between what is available, what is acceptable to parents, and what is best suited to the child's needs.

Management of behaviour

Behavioural management is based on classical and operant conditioning. Good behaviour is rewarded and undesirable behaviour eliminated by teaching alternative behaviours. Vigorous exercise can be effective in reducing behavioural problems such as aggressiveness and self-injurious behaviour. Parents, teachers and caregivers need continual encouragement to specify desirable behaviour rather than proscribing undesirable behaviour. Saying, "Don't do ..." is much more likely to be heard as "John do ..." Schemes to teach social rules, especially those for adolescents, can be helpful.

The aim is to develop a "library" of rules to cover most contingencies, with parental recognition that there will be times when they will be inadequate.

Vocational training

A special interest can become the basis for an occupation. As autism is a lifelong disorder individualised support is required in work placement and training. This becomes the dominant parental concern as the prospect of school draws to a close.

Pharmacotherapy

Medication has only a small role in the management of autism and should be symptom targeted, as there is no specific medication available. Drugs should be used as an adjunct to psychosocial approaches.

Seizures should be treated with anticonvulsant therapy. When depression or obsessional and ritualistic behaviours are distressing serotonin selective reuptake inhibitors (SSRIs) should be tried. SSRIs are also helpful, if introduced slowly, for disruptive behaviour. Neuroleptics (for example risperidone) may be of value in breaking vicious cycles in the aggressive adolescent who has failed to respond to SSRIs. Lithium and anticonvulsant medication may be helpful in controlling major mood swings, especially in adolescence, as well as for treatment resistant aggression.

Self-injurious behaviour may require one or more of the above therapies.

Prognosis and outcome

Avoidance of physical contact improves with time but reciprocal play with age-related peers remains unchanged in most. During adolescence there may be increased aggression and mood swings, but these difficulties diminish in later adolescence.

The child's cognitive level and language impairment are the strongest prediction of outcome. Those with performance IQ below 50 will remain severely handicapped and dependent on others. If a child has a normal non-verbal intelligence and useful communicative language by 5 years of age, there is a 50% chance of a reasonable level of social adjustment in adult life. Most will require support both in the workplace and in daily living. Parents mostly make adjustments slowly and in piecemeal fashion. Helping them in this process requires sensitivity, patience and respect for their perseverance.

Asperger's syndrome

Asperger's syndrome is generally considered to be on a continuum with autism and autistic-like conditions. However, it is unclear whether it represents autism with normal intelligence (so called "high functioning autism") or whether it has a specific cognitive profile. It is characterised by:

- Severe impairment in reciprocal social interaction
- An all absorbing narrow interest taken to an extreme
- Speech and language problems
- Non-verbal communication problems
- Motor clumsiness.

Epidemiology

Asperger's syndrome is approximately 10 times more common in boys than girls. The prevalence is at least 3 per 1000 children born. It is usually diagnosed between the ages of 7 and 10 years as a result of restricted interests, motor clumsiness, and lack of empathy. However, the diagnosis may be overlooked until the child enters high school or it may never be made.

Aetiology

There is frequently a relative with similar problems implying that genetic factors are important. At least half of all children with Asperger's syndrome have a parent with the same (or similar) condition. It can also accompany tuberous sclerosis, neurofibromatosis, fragile X syndrome, and perinatal brain damage.

Clinical features

Asperger's syndrome presents as social and motor ineptitude with dominating preoccupations and an odd mode of communication.

Features of the social skill impairment include a reduced interest or ability to socialise, a reduced appreciation of social cues, and in some socially and emotionally inappropriate behaviour.

The speech and language problems include delayed development of language, superficially perfect expressive language, a tendency to literalness, and an unusual tone. There are also difficulties in making sense of others and using language appropriately, despite a knowledge of the words. Speech therapists often refer to the speech as a "semantic-pragmatic disorder".

Non-verbal communication problems include limited use of gestures, clumsy/gauche body language, and reduced, inappropriate or stiff facial expressions. Group activities, especially rough games, are stressful. Other features include obstinacy and aggressive outbursts when these children are under pressure to conform, emotional detachment, rigidity, and marked sensitivity.

Curiously, despite average intelligence, they may still have learning problems and some display antisocial behaviour, particularly during adolescence.

A particularly prominent feature of this disorder is the inability to reflect on other people's "inner world" (moods, thoughts, wishes, beliefs, and feelings). This is not as prominent as in autism, as some reflection on another's needs can usually be attained if pushed, and some capacity usually develops with age. Additionally, even when there is good cognitive capacity to consider another person's needs this may not be carried out in a real life setting.

The child can often attain any individual social skill in isolation but finds the whole task of relating difficult to sustain.

Differential diagnosis

Many of the children have associated attentional difficulties and obsessional features making the diagnosis of attention

Table 16.1 Asperger's syndrome: differential diagnosis with autism

Autism	Asperger's syndrome
Social aloofness	Social oddity
Absent language or marked language abnormality	Subtle qualitative language differences
Usually no motor incoordination	Clumsy with a lack of fluidity of movement
Behaviour dominated by repetitive activities	Speech and behaviour dominated by repetitive themes and interests
Friends and relatives left in no doubt that an autistic child does not understand social situations and intimate relationships	Friends and relatives left uncertain, frustrated or bewildered as to what they do and do not understand

deficit hyperactivity disorder and obsessive compulsive disorder common. However, their rigidity, and misunderstanding of social cues are frequently confused with antisocial behaviour. When placed under academic or social pressure many become very distressed with a disproportionate number going on to develop psychotic illnesses in later adolescence.

The differential diagnosis with autism presents a constant dilemma (Table 16.1).

The following investigations are recommended:

- Opthalmology assessment
- Audiological testing
- Chromosomal analysis
- Psychometric assessment—there are typically relatively lower results on comprehension, picture arrangement, and similarities.

Treatment

Education

It is important to support parents and inform them about the disorder and the help available with education and social problems. Help will be especially needed during the transition through early adolescence.

Parents are encouraged to:

- Sustain an approximate but regular routine, which makes life predictable
- Introduce change slowly, systematically and regularly where possible
- Pace academic progress on social/emotional development rather than intellectual development.

Parents should be discouraged from:

- Coercive confrontation over difficult behaviour
- Forcing socialisation
- Unqualified accommodation to the child's rigidity and preoccupations.

Management depends on identifying what the child can and cannot change and how the parents and clinician can determine this. Additionally it is important for the parent to understand the child as much as possible so that the child may subsequently understand the parent. Parents and other family members have often inadvertently accommodated to the difficulties of the child by adapting their daily routine. Asperger's syndrome is a chronic disability, which is usually more socially than intellectually impairing, and consequently the presence of the disorder may be less obvious.

Prognosis

Many manage fairly well in adult life in terms of education, employment, and marriage. However some may become depressed and make suicidal attempts and others carry out criminal offences. They may wish for closer relationships as they grow into adulthood but find them difficult to attain and their inflexibility makes the sustaining of a job difficult. Much depends upon the adaptability and acceptance of people close to them.

Rett's syndrome

This disorder occurs in girls, aged 5–30 months, manifested by a loss of hand skills and verbal communication. This is

Table 16.2 Important differentiating features between autism and Rett's syndrome

Rett's syndrome	Autism
Girls only	Boys more than girls
Always low IQ	Variable IQ
Regression of all milestones	Usually only partial and short-lived regression
Inconsolable crying and lack of facial expression	—
Lose speech	Slow to develop speech
Seizures early in life	Seizures occur in 25% of adolescents
Deceleration in head growth (normal circumference at birth)	Head circumference larger than average
Hypotonia then hypertonia (broad based gait)	Gait and tone usually normal
Shortening of fourth metacarpal, metatarsal and ulnar bone	No shortening of bones
Truncal rocking, hand wringing, clapping or tapping in midline of the body	Central and non-central flapping
Hyperventilation	No hyperventilation

accompanied by social impairment, stereotypical hand wringing or clapping in the midline, hyperventilation, and truncal ataxia. With increasing age there is further motor and intellectual decline. Rett's syndrome has been described as a dementia with autistic features but is probably more accurately viewed as social and communication skills in keeping with their very low mental age.

Table 16.2 displays important differentiating features between autism and Rett's syndrome .

Treatment

There is no known treatment for Rett's syndrome but as much support as possible should be provided for child and family.

Prognosis

There is progressive deterioration in cognitive and motor function, loss of purposive hand movements, the emergence of seizures, and neuromuscular impairment.

Conclusion

Autistic spectrum disorders show a wide diversity in the severity of impairment in the social, communication and flexibility domains. Many children suffering from mental retardation will have some autistic features and in practice it is often difficult to decide if they have an additional diagnosis of autistic spectrum disorder. In managing autistic disorders a multidisciplinary approach that focuses on developing skill deficits and provides support for the parents offers the best outcomes.

Reference

Rutter M. Infantile autism. In: Shaffer D, Erdhardt A, Greenhill L, eds. *A Clinician's guide to child psychiatry*. New York: Free Press, 1985:48–78.

Further reading

Bailey A, Philips W, Rutter M. Autism—towards an integration of clinical, genetic, neuropsychological and neurobiological perspectives. *Journal of Child Psychology and Psychiatry and Allied Disciplines* 1996;**37**:89–126.

Gillberg C. *Clinical child neuropsychiatry*. Cambridge: Cambridge University Press, 1995:chapter 6.

Kerr A. Annotation: Rett syndrome—recent progress and implications for research and clinical practice. *Journal of Child Psychology and Psychiatry* 2002;**43**:277–87.

Lord C, Rutter M. Autism and pervasive developmental disorders. In: Taylor E, Hersov L, eds. *Child and adult psychiatry. Modern approaches*. Oxford: Blackwell Science, 1994:569–93.

Volkmar F, Cook E, Pomeroy J, Realmuto G, Tanguay P. Practice parameters for the assessment and treatment of autism and other pervasive development disorders, 1999. *Journal of the American Academy of Child and Adolescent Psychiatry* 1999;**38**:32S–54S.

17: Neurodevelopmental disorders

Introduction

Overall, at least 5% of school age children in the general population show clear signs of neuropsychiatric disorder. Between 25% and 50% of all consultations in child and adolescent psychiatry can be defined as neuropsychiatric problems. This chapter concentrates on delirium, dementia, psychological aspects of epilepsy, head injury, and frontal lobe disorders, together with a general perspective on any disorder involving the brain. Children with neurodevelopmental problems are not fundamentally different from most children with psychiatric disorder. The overlap with the full range of psychiatric disorder is extensive.

Clinical assessment

The experience of a troubled brain

Children, especially small children, often have difficulty articulating the location of their pain or the bodily source of their distress. When the brain is affected, the different types of child presentation may camouflage the source of distress for a considerable length of time.

Symptoms

Troubled brains are experienced as:

- *"I feel all mixed up."* Confusion and bewilderment in the case of delirium.
- *"People keep asking me but I don't remember anything."* Unexplained gaps in experience in the case of seizures, traumatic brain injury, delirium, and transient amnesic disorders.

- *"I can't stay awake."* Inability to stay awake, go to sleep or untroubled sleep in the sleep disorders and parasomnias.
- *"They just won't leave me alone."* Other people being experienced as unduly annoying and provocative. Children with episodic dyscontrol of aggression and Asperger's syndrome perceive others as provoking them.
- *"Movements that keep happening even when I don't want them to."* Tics, dystonias, choreas and ballistic movements may all be experienced as "invading" the body or ignored as if they were not occurring at all.
- *"Everyone else seems worried about me."* Conversion disorders can worry the children who are afflicted with them but a significant minority do not trouble their owners at all.
- *"Everyone is smarter than me."* Intellectual impairment leaves many children feeling "at the bottom of the heap". Paradoxically, this feeling is likely to be worse the milder the impairment.
- *"I don't know."* Disorders of declarative memory, generally due to hippocampal damage, leave the child user of memory without any confidence or conviction of knowing even if it subsequently becomes clear that they do know.
- *"It's all too hard."* Cognitive slowing, cognitive deficit and motivational loss are all common in a wide range of brain disorders. This is especially so where the frontal systems are involved. Outwardly, it may look like the child has a lack of concern, care and absence of enthusiasm and stickability. Internally it often feels that what is being asked for is all too hard.

Assessing inconsistent patterns of symptoms and signs

Adaptation to the environment is the work of the brain. When the brain does not work properly it usually does so incompletely. Different situations, people, times of the day and tasks will produce very different results. Partial maladaptation and differing responses are often called "inconsistency". Patterns are helpful but there is much more variability in medical disorder than is commonly acknowledged. Inconsistent symptoms and signs may be due to organic disorder:

- Exercise induced dystonia disappears on rest.
- Tics and tremor reduce, and often disappear completely, with sleep.
- Memory disorders may vary on the task being tested. For example in so called declarative memory disorders the child does not think they "know" even though they do. Some children show that they know even though they do not know that they know.
- The body and brain are not always consistent with our testing techniques.
- Inconsistency of physical signs has to be gross to reassure us that it is not biologically based. Unless gross, it is suggestive but not pathognomonic of psychological disorder.

Assessing the degree of voluntary control

Tics can be suppressed for a time, concentration can be mustered, and pain can be ignored. There is even evidence that in some seizure disorders a voluntary component exists. I may be able to jump over a hurdle in panic when my life is at stake but I may not be able to jump over 10 hurdles as part of a race every day of my life. "He can do it when he wants to!" is a worrying assertion. Psychological components to problems are under less voluntary control than is often imagined. Mood disorders, psychosis and most forms of psychological disorder are as painful, distressing and as involuntary as most medical disorders.

Defining the symptomatic presentation

The ability of children to relate, to adapt in response to ordinary, everyday tasks and to perform the more demanding processes of planning and organising their futures are the critical elements of the assessment.

Putting into words what *we can and cannot do* in an examination with a child or a family often illuminates as much as the presence of any particular ability, disability, or clinical phenomenon.

Investigation

Most diagnoses are made on history and only supported by investigation. Testing of particular hypotheses is much more likely to yield meaningful results. Even negative results have a function and provide important reassurance on what is not happening.

There is only a modest relationship between structure and function for most current measures. Marginally positive tests of any sort may be particularly misleading. A child may have epilepsy with a normal EEG. A child may have an abnormal EEG but not have epilepsy. This does not mean the EEG is useless but rather that it is limited and interpreted in light of the clinical picture by an experienced paediatric neurologist. Epilepsy remains a clinical diagnosis based on history and examination. An abnormal EEG alone does not constitute epilepsy.

CT and MRI will generally delineate structure rather than function. By contrast, single photon emission (SPECT) and positron emission tomography (PET) delineate function rather than structure. Neuropsychological testing will delineate function sometimes more accurately than all other current methods. It is important to separate out what phenomena the child exhibits, what tests are abnormal, and then to ask the separate but critical question : "How likely is it that the clinical picture is connected to the abnormality of test function?"

Testing must be reviewed critically and within the context of the child's case details. Even within a very short time period histories and reported results can become distorted. It is always valuable to verify previous results to avoid "Chinese whispers". The results of tests upon which the future of an individual depends should not be reported over the phone by someone who did not do the investigation. When results are critical for the future of an individual take care to get the true result even if it takes a little longer.

Making a diagnosis

Having a psychological disorder does not protect against, and in fact increases the possibility of, a medical disorder.

Having a brain disorder increases the likelihood of a psychological disorder. Different environments will draw out different symptoms depending upon the nature of the underlying deficit, especially early on in the disorder.

Global or focal impairment of function?

When approaching problems of brain function it is best to begin by asking simple questions and making very obvious observations. Is the whole brain affected, a few parts, or just one? Is the brain able to do most of its normal tasks? It is possible that a very critical component of the brain is damaged, affecting the whole brain.

Dysfunction, damage, and decline

If the whole of the brain has a problem, we need to ask further very basic questions. Is the problem due to the brain struggling (dysfunction) and therefore potentially correctable? Is the problem due to a condition which is reflecting the brain in global damage (non-correctable) or global dying (progressive damage)?

Single episode or recurrent

If the problem involves the whole brain, is it a new or recurrent problem?

If new is it likely to recur? If recurrent what is the level of recovery after each episode?

With these questions in mind we turn to consider the psychiatric disorders arising from altered brain function.

Disorders

Delirium—a brain under threat

Delirium is the fluctuating clouding of consciousness that affects the ability of children to respond appropriately to their surroundings. This is usually due to an underlying medical disorder but sometimes the cause remains unknown.

193

Delerious children are not so drowsy as to be almost unrousable or totally unresponsive as in stupor and coma. Delirium usually, but not always, develops over a period of hours or days. The difficulties are not explicable alone by the presence of seizures, dementia, or memory disorders. Many other analogous and related terms to delirium are used, such as confusional state, encephalopathic state, acute brain syndrome, and toxic encephalopathy.

Aetiology

Possible causes include:

- Hypoxia
- Hypoglycaemia
- Systemic infection
- CNS infection
- Polypharmacy, especially with anticholinergics, anticonvulsants, and psychotropics
- Substance abuse or withdrawal
- Accidental and non-accidental overdose
- Medications—steroids, anticholinergics, lithium, all neurotropics and psychotropics, and anticholinesterases
- Inflammation
- Radiation
- Raised or fluctuating intracranial pressures
- CNS trauma
- Mitochondrial disorder
- High stimulation non-periodised environments like intensive care units
- Low stimulation isolated environments like detainment centres for youth offenders, single rooms in busy wards, and orthopaedic immobilisation.

Clinical presentation

Someone else is troubled Children with delirium rarely identify their own problem except by volunteering hallucinations. Others become worried for them due to changes in appearance, behaviour, speech content or process, perceptions, affect, social interactions, or cognitions.

Conditions confused with delirium

- The functional psychoses—especially bipolar disorder
- Kleine–Levin syndrome
- Peripubertal psychosis
- Menstrually related hypersomnia
- Dementia and more limited neurocognitive decline
- Akinetic mutism.

Treatment

The treatment of delirium involves a judgement as to whether the delirium is mild and/or predominantly hypoactive or severe and/or predominantly hyperactive. The milder the delirium and the more hypoactive the more helpful is the increase in sensory stimulation, reality orienting information and consideration of dopamine agonist medications. The basic strategy is to increase arousal. The more severe and the more predominant the hyperactivity the more likely is the child or teenager to benefit from increasing the depth of the delirium by sedation and using dopamine antagonists. The presence of mutism, extrapyramidal signs and dysautonomia will also favour dopamine agonists, while hallucinations, delusions and incoherence of thought will favour dopamine antagonists. Where the picture is mixed with hyperactive and hypoactive elements and severe, it is best to proceed with a sedating dopamine antagonist initially.

A stable airway must be maintained. If this is particularly difficult transfer to an intensive care unit. The vast majority will be maintained with special nursing and frequent, repeated nursing observations.

Prognosis

This is dependent upon cause. Where delirium has been deep, prolonged and associated with signs of encephalopathy, the possibility of intellectual deficit has to be considered likely. Experience suggests that this is usually less than 15 IQ points but bigger losses do occur. As with head injury, recovery may occur up to 2 years later, but most recovery occurs in the first 12 months.

> **Box 17.1 More frequent conditions giving rise to progressive dementia**
>
> - Leigh's disease and other mitochondrial (including MELAS and Alpers' disease) disorders
> - Rett's disorder
> - Metachromatic leukodystrophy
> - Subacute sclerosing panencephalitis (SSPE)
> - Batten's disease
> - Adrenoleukodystrophy
> - Mucopolysaccharidoses
> - Niemann–Pick disease
> - Pelizaeus–Merzbacher disease
> - Tay–Sachs and Tay–Sachs variant
> - Multiple sclerosis

Dementia—a brain in decline

Definition

Dementia in childhood involves the pervasive and progressive loss of already attained developmental skills. This usually reduces the child's subsequent developmental trajectory and generally, but not always, leads to death. The condition is not explicable in terms of acute drug toxicity or the other causes of delirium.

Epidemiology

The incidence is unknown but likely to be between 5 and 15 per 100 000.

Aetiology

There are over 600 possible diseases, syndromes and conditions that are known to be able to give rise to dementia in childhood. The most common conditions are listed in Box 17.1.

Clinical presentation

The varieties of presentation will depend upon the developmental stage of the child and the nature of the neuropathology.

In infancy, loss of fixing and following with the eyes and alteration in the quality of cry might be the only signs of regression. Toddlers may lose already accomplished skills of walking and speech and develop an autistic picture. The school age child may develop visual difficulties, learning and behaviour problems, loss of writing skills and a drop off in school function with social withdrawal. Seizures are a possible presenting feature at any age.

Assessment and investigation

Once the serious possibility of dementia has been invoked it is critical to involve a paediatric neurologist with whom investigation can be planned strategically. However, most of the time, dementia as a differential diagnosis will be in the "less likely but needs to be considered and excluded" category.

Six key questions need to be answered:

1. Is there a definite history of sustained skill loss or merely a short term falling off of trajectory?
2. Are there any neurological features to the presentation such as seizures, ataxia, deterioration in vision or weakness which might give a clue as to the nature of the disorder?
3. Is there a family history that is suggestive of one of the dementing conditions?
4. How might the stage of development affect the presentation of the disorder?
5. What is the current impact on the family of the disorder and the threat associated with the disorder?
6. Are any of the siblings similarly affected?

All children with suspected dementia should have full neurological examination, neurological investigations, and neuropsychometric assessment.

Differential diagnosis

This includes:

- Severe and profound depression
- Pervasive refusal syndrome

- Cerebral tumours
- Schizophrenia
- Side effects of medication
- Somatoform disorder
- Factitious disorder.

Treatment

This includes:

- Ascertaining the aetiology
- Treating the psychiatric symptoms
- Supporting the family
- Appropriate educational placement.

Prognosis

Most dementia is irreversible although hypothyroidism, vitamin B_{12} deficiency, hydrocephalus and the hyperphenylalanaemias are all potentially reversible, and many of the neurometabolic disorders which now result in dementia may, in time, be treatable.

Nor does all dementia lead inexorably onto death, although life will be foreshortened in almost all cases to some degree due to the complications of intellectual impairment and seizures. Some dementias progress to a certain point then plateau.

Epilepsy—a storm in the brain

Introduction

The absolute rate of psychiatric disorder is more than double that of other chronic medical disorders not involving the central nervous system, and as much as five times higher than in the normal population. Not all epilepsy increases the risk of comorbid psychological impairment, and much psychiatric disorder attributed to epilepsy is unrelated and better understood in the light of environmental factors alone. The role of epilepsy in contributing to psychiatric disorder has been variously formulated as:

- *Coincidental.* They happen by chance to occur together.
- *Cophenomenal.* Caused by the same brain pathology that gave rise to the epilepsy.
- *Threshold reducing.* The types of disorder are not unique in type or variety but are increased in frequency and induced with less environmental stimulus.
- *Lesion specific.* Depending upon the location of the epilepsy, the environmental demand, and whether the lesion is seizure active or not.

Clinical presentations

The child with psychiatric disorder who happens to have epilepsy There is compelling evidence that children with epilepsy have a lower threshold to all psychiatric disorders and that this exceeds the vulnerability created by chronic medical disorder not involving the central nervous system. In general, where the epilepsy has been stabilised this should be managed by establishing the psychiatric treatment and then recalibrating the anticonvulsants.

The child whose principal problem is epilepsy but has associated psychiatric disorder There are several forms of associations:

- *Ictal behaviour abnormality.* The important feature of these uncommon seizures is the prominent psychiatric features. Behaviourally bizarre seizures with complicated behavioural sequences, usually involving the frontal lobes, may be misdiagnosed as hysteria. They may last for several minutes, but occasionally in excess of an hour. These episodes are characterised by behavioural complexity rather than ideational or perceptual distortion. Other ictal abnormalities include aura related violence, running, or stereotyped behaviour such as laughing, crying, and automatisms.
- *Interictal behaviour disorder.* Disinhibited, overactive, easily distractible behaviour which is aggressive and disruptive is common.
- *Iatrogenic comorbidity.* Anxiety, depression, disruptive disorders including attention deficit hyperactivity disorder, psychosis, delirium, pseudodementia and rarely dementia have all been documented in relation to anticonvulsant medication. These have reduced with the reduced use of barbiturates and phenytoin but remain more frequent

with the benzodiazepines, vigabatrin, gabapentin, and topiramate.

- *Misery and helplessness.* Cognitive slowing, social stigma and fear of seizures corrodes self-esteem and restricts social confidence and activity. Illness education, reduction of inappropriate academic demands and steady social rehabilitation all reduce the assumption of helplessness as a posture toward their illness.
- *Ictal psychosis.* This rare disorder can be very dramatic with sudden onset, intense paranoia, automatisms, and even violence or self-injury. Consciousness is clouded, emotions fearful or angry, and thoughts are inaccessible. They may last for seconds to minutes though may be prolonged into hours or even rarely days. They are usually frontotemporal in origin.

Assessment and investigation

Assessment and investigation should be done hand in hand with a paediatric neurologist or the available paediatrician. Videotelemetry and ambulatory monitoring are often helpful. However, many of these children promptly stop having seizures and episodes on coming into hospital. This should not be taken as evidence of hysteria. The key elements on history include:

- *Age of onset.* In general the earlier the onset the worse the prognosis and the worse the behavioural impact and the demands upon family adjustment.
- *Impact on development.* If impairment of function is profound behavioural impact and demands upon the family may be paradoxically less.
- *The nature of the behavioural and emotional disorder.* Depression may be sudden and severe. Disruptive disorders are particularly problematic when there is a degree of frontal disinhibition associated with aggression. Ictal psychotic episodes are often extremely stereotyped.
- *The type of seizure.* Complex partial seizures with variable seizure types are much more likely to be associated with psychopathology than uncomplicated absence or tonic clonic seizures.
- *The best level of functioning* to which the child might return. Sometimes it is necessary to go back as far as 2 years but usually function in the last 12 months is most relevant.

- *The family adjustment.* Childhood epilepsy acts as a chronic cumulative stressor on parents and the rate of parental psychopathology rises with each year from illness onset.

Investigation

This should include:

- Daily sleep, behaviour, mood and seizure charts—all enable more accurate decision making than vague retrospective generalisations.
- Educational assessment—specific learning difficulties, concentration and cognitive processing difficulties.
- Psychometric assessment—when no paediatric neuro-psychologist is available a sound thoughtful general psychometric assessment is often worth more than a highly speculative and inexpert neuropsychological report.
- A review of all medications and where appropriate serum levels are essential.
- A review of all previous investigations and histories of previous admissions often reveals forgotten but nevertheless relevant information.

Treatment

This involves judicious use of medication for both the epilepsy and the psychiatric disorder (see chapter 25), ensuring that any medication does not aggravate the situation, parental support (see chapter 22), and occasionally cognitive behavioural therapy (see chapter 24).

Prognosis

The prognosis is quite variable and difficult to predict.

Pseudoseizures—a brain in the storm

Pseudoseizures mimic seizures but are not epileptic in origin. However the most likely child to have a pseudoseizure is one who also has epileptic seizures. Pseudoseizures are generally more prolonged than seizures, less injurious, associated with persisting clarity of consciousness, and are less controlled by medication. They may also be distinguished by the fact that following real seizures there is generally a postictal rise in prolactin.

Pseudoseizures generally occur in shy, sensitive and vulnerable children and are triggered by such factors as stress, need for caring, or as a way out of a difficult predicament.

Treatment

This includes:

- Recognition and management of the major role stress can play in any seizure disorder.
- Avoidance of stigmatisation.
- Promotion of healthy activity in regular but manageable amounts.
- Anxiety management for carers.
- Provision of a structured day that is not overwhelmingly demanding, competitive, or perfectionistic.
- Provision of affection and attention to be given regularly, predictably, and not in response to the seizures alone.
- Establishment of a clear problem solving approach to predicaments the child faces.

Prognosis

When pseudoseizures are managed as a common and understandable complication of epilepsy they are usually brought under control rapidly and easily, provided the general approach is supportive and the causes are addressed. Occasionally longstanding family pathology will prevent resolution and the pseudoseizures become intractable.

A traumatised brain

Introduction

The following general features should be considered:

- Head injuries are the most common causes of traumatised brains in childhood.

- Road traffic accidents are the most common cause of severe head injury.
- All injury is more common in boys than girls.
- Sadly, parental abuse remains a significant minority cause, especially in the under threes.

Closed head injuries threaten global brain function through powerful sheering forces, laceration and contusion contrecoup injuries especially affecting the temporal lobes. Loss of consciousness with post-traumatic amnesia is the rule.

Open head injuries have less contrecoup damage, more local damage with the possibility of infection, and post-traumatic epilepsy.

Aetiology

The relationship between psychopathology and head injury is more complex than is at first apparent. Head injury, or indeed any injury, is more likely when parenting is compromised, reckless, or abusive. Head injury is also more likely when children's behaviour is unpredictable, impulsive, heedless of consequence, and lacking in vigilance. Conditions such as attention deficit hyperactivity disorder make injury more likely. Other factors include substance abuse and intellectual impairment.

Clinical presentations

The neglect–disruption cycle Exhausted parents, perhaps with limited resources, tend to pay attention more to their brain damaged children when they are disruptive. The disruptive behaviour further exhausts the parents, who then neglect and ignore their children until they are disruptive yet again, setting up a cycle of reinforced disruption and diminishing recovery periods.

The narrowed stimulus window Most children become overwhelmed, distressed or disruptive if there is too little or too much stimulus. In traumatic brain injury this window between boredom and stimulus overload is narrowed. The child is always in need of something to do but never too much. This means that parents require a level of vigilance and planning that is usually unnecessary in normal children. As a consequence parents become overregulated with little time to themselves. Regular, planned, non-crisis driven respite is necessary.

Acquired intellectual disability Children who have been developing normally, who have already gained important emotional, social and cognitive skills, and who have their trajectory altered may evoke very different responses to those who had lower trajectories from birth. They may also have bigger islands of preservation of function.

Frontal lobe syndromes See below.

The lowered threshold for any disorder Over and above pre-existing disorder, specific traumatic focal disorder and generalised intellectual disability, there is a lowering of threshold to emotional and disruptive disorders in the presence of environmental risk factors or precipitants. These disorders, which are often not qualitatively different to those in non-traumatised young people, arise more easily in response to environmental stressors.

Assessment and investigation

While EEG and MRI are clearly critical, developmental and neuropsychological testing will offer much more functional information for serial assessment and plotting of altered functional trajectory.

Treatment and education

Education with a view to explaining behaviours, shaping expectations and reducing unhelpful responses from parents, siblings and teachers is the mainstay of psychological care.

Prognosis

- Most cognitive recovery occurs in the first year after injury with further minor gains over 2–3 years.
- Unusually, recovery can occur up to 5 years after injury.

- Equally some impairment may not become apparent until later when expected developmental advances fail to occur. This applies particularly in those with injuries in the first 2 years of life.
- Those with post-traumatic amnesias lasting greater than 3 weeks are likely to have persistent cognitive deficit.
- Those with severe head injuries are likely to have psychiatric disorder (> 50%) and this effect does not diminish within the first 2 years.
- Those who have psychosocial adversity and severe disorder have a disproportionate rate of new disorder arising from the interaction.

Conclusion

Traumatic brain injury is an important cause of cognitive and emotional impairment, especially where the injury is closed, severe, associated with contrecoup, prolonged post-traumatic amnesia, and psychosocial adversity. It is surprising how often severe head injury is ignored when the behavioural problems are being considered 1–2 years later. It is also surprising how much is attributed to minor head injuries at other times.

Frontal lobe syndromes (a brain without brakes, and sometimes an accelerator too!)

The frontal lobes form part of those brain systems that anticipate, plan and prepare for the future. They inhibit unwanted, inappropriate or unacceptable responses. They enable thinking about the business in hand while manipulating possible responses.

Children with frontal lobe difficulties who have little response to social disapproval may appear disruptive or antisocial. Children who have planning and other executive difficulties, and who are overactive and have problems with working memory, may be indistinguishable from those with attention deficit disorder and hyperactivity.

Those who are apathetic, disinterested, emotionally labile and more or less mute, may appear depressed.

Aetiology

The range of possible injuries to the frontal lobes is large. Traumatic brain injury is the most common, but other conditions include encephalitis, meningitis, neoplastic infiltration, toxic gas inhalation, anoxia, degenerative and inflammatory causes such as cerebral lupus.

Clinical presentation

There are five main presentations:

1. The inert apathetic child who cannot get started and has difficulty keeping going.
2. The socially garrulous and disinhibited child who is difficult to contain, socially inappropriate, and emotionally "incontinent".
3. The child who presents as if with attention deficit hyperactivity disorder but is more disturbed and less responsive to treatment.
4. The perseverative child who has a limited repertoire of responses to stress.
5. The unempathic and episodically aggressive child, whose violence can be lethal.

Aetiology

Head injury, infarction of brain tissue, infection, neoplasm and degenerative disorder may all give rise to a frontal lobe syndrome.

Assessment and investigation

In most cases the history will be the most helpful contributor to diagnostic decision making. Sequential school reports are often helpful in documenting change in social behaviour.

Neuropsychological testing can be helpful in cases where the syndrome is more subtle and the impairment less overt. However, frontal neuropsychological tests of executive function can be unproductive and misleading even where the clinical syndrome is quite blatant. Single photon emission CT

(SPECT) scanning may reveal inflammatory causes, EEG may reveal seizures, MRI may define structural damage, and magnetic resonance (MR) spectroscopy may reveal evidence of neuronal breakdown suggestive of neurodegenerative disorder.

Treatment

Simple explanations of the underlying pathology and the connection between brain function and behaviour reduce uncertainty.

The tendency to normalise quite unusual behaviour for a particular child has to be resisted. The long term personality and behaviour of the child and the change that has occurred are emphasised and the invisible disability made overt.

Parents are encouraged to take on frontal functions on behalf of the child in the short term, while it is being clarified to what extent this will need to done in the long term. School will need to be similarly informed and structured supportive frameworks will be necessary both in the classroom and in the playground.

Helping everyone move from a moral framework of understanding the child to a medical understanding will be critical. There is almost always someone who finds it difficult not to see the child as "plain naughty" or in adolescence, "antisocial".

Dopamine agonists, tricyclics and the antipsychotics may all be considered.

Prognosis

Where the underlying pathology is acute and treatable the prognosis may be guardedly optimistic. However, chronic disorder usually requires a decision for the environment, usually the parents, to assume the role of the frontal lobes in the child's and young person's life. Once having assumed this role it is difficult to relinquish.

Conclusion

Children with neurodevelopmental problems act as chronic cumulative stressors upon their environment, especially their parents and siblings. This field requires a close working relationship with neurologists, neuropsychologists, and general paediatric clinicians. Modern best practice demands that biological, psychological and contextual factors are all considered within assessment and treatment. Parental counselling, family therapy and cognitive behaviour therapy can all help in coping with neurodevelopmental problems. They may not remove the disorder but they can ameliorate the situation.

Further reading

Coffey CE, Brumback RA. *Textbook of pediatric neuropsychiatry.* Washington: American Psychiatric Association Press, 1998.
Gillberg C. *Clinical child neuropsychiatry.* Cambridge: Cambridge University Press, 1995.
Harris J. *Developmental neuropsychiatry,* Vols 1, 2. Oxford: Oxford University Press, 1995.
Nunn KP. Neuropsychiatry in childhood: residential treatment. In: Green J, Jacobs B, eds. *In-patient child psychiatry—modern practice, research and the future.* London: Routledge, 1998:258–84.
Nunn KP, Williams K, Ouvrier R. The Australian Childhood Dementia Study. *European Child and Adolescent Psychiatry* 2002;11:63–70.
Volkmar FR. *Psychoses and pervasive developmental disorders in childhood and adolescence.* Washington: American Psychiatric Press and the American Academy of Child and Adolescent Psychiatry, 1996.

18: The maltreated child

Introduction

Maltreatment occurs in many forms including emotional, physical and sexual abuse, and neglect. Each component of abuse has its own spectrum of severity, complexity, and specific pathological features. All clinicians require an understanding of the nature of maltreatment in all its forms and the principles of first line management. In this chapter basic strategies for assessment and management are outlined.

The spectra of maltreatment

Child maltreatment and parenting capacity are inextricably linked in that poor parenting can imperceptibly merge with abuse. For example, accidents may occur as a result of lapses in the usual protection given to a child. Neglect, i.e. parenting with failure of basic provision of care and protection from harm, generally occurs more consistently whilst abuse may be either impulsive or deliberate. Although the different forms of abuse and maltreatment are discussed separately for the sake of clarity, the presence of one form of maltreatment is often associated with another.

Physical abuse

Introduction

There are many definitions of physical abuse (sometimes called non-accidental injury, or NAI), most of which involve injury to soft tissues such as skin, eyes, ears and internal organs together with damage to ligaments and bones. Punching, slapping, whipping, scalding, burning, starving, cutting and shaking are among the most common. Central nervous system damage remains the most permanent legacy for many children. When death from NAI occurs it is usually in the first year of life.

Although NAI can occur in any setting such as school, day care and special nursery facilities, it is most common within the family, including at the hands of a step-parent or common-law partner of the biological mother. While NAI can occur in otherwise well functioning families under exceptional stress, severe or repetitive NAI usually reflects longer term parenting difficulties. One of the barriers to diagnosis can be the belief and wish that no one could do this to their child or, indeed to any child.

Diagnosis

The following factors should raise the suspicion of physical abuse:

- Delay or failure in seeking medical attention.
- Vague, inconsistent and often variable historical details of the injury.
- Repeated presentations with injuries.
- Parental failure to be sensitive to the needs of their child, even during the interview.
- Hostility to the interviewer asking even basic and reasonable questions.
- Wanting to take the child home before completing the assessment or obtaining treatment.
- Lack of any guilt that their children are injured, sometimes with blame for the children themselves, or their siblings.
- Parental attribution to their child of abilities and attitudes in advance of, and out of keeping with, their developmental capacities and known behaviour.

Key features during the examination

- Child looks sad, miserable or frightened. In extreme cases this may take the form of "frozen watchfulness". In older children a reluctance to talk about how they were injured is particularly worrying. In other cases a child will simply say "Mummy did it!"or "they hit me because I was bad".

- Children may disclose away from the parent how they received the injuries. It is imperative where abuse is suspected that an interview in the absence of parents takes place.
- The actual examination may show a child reluctant to use an arm or leg, fingertip bruising from forceful grabbing and gripping of the child, cigarette burns, lash marks (linear marks with tram-lining), retinal haemorrhages, and a torn frenulum. Growth charts may indicate failure to thrive.
- Irritability, vomiting, difficulties in breathing, decreasing levels of consciousness and retinal haemorrhages after a reportedly trivial incident in the infant are NAI until proven otherwise, and constitute a medical and surgical emergency.

Key features in investigation

Fractures   Investigation may reveal multiple bruises and old or new fractures, especially in those under 3 years of age where alternative explanations are less likely. The following are all highly suggestive of NAI: single fractures with multiple bruises, multiple fractures at different stages of healing, unexplained rib and skull fractures, fractures separating the ends of long bones as a chip or plate ("corner fractures"), marked healing growth under the membrane around bones (periosteal reaction) where bleeding has occurred, spiral midshaft fractures, and complex skull fractures.

Fractures less likely to be significant are single fractures, linear and unseparated parietal fractures of the skull, simple long bone fractures, and clavicular fractures.

Head injury   Accidental intracranial injury in infancy is rare. Head injury and abdominal injuries are the main cause of death in NAI. Estimates of NAI causes of serious intracranial injury during the first year of life exceed 90%. Skull fractures, subdural haematomas, subarachnoid haemorrhage, cerebral oedema, haematomas between scalp and skull, growing fractures of the skull (because of cerebral swelling) and traumatic hair loss are all seen in NAI. Subdurals can often arise in the absence of a skull fracture secondary to violent shaking, usually to stop the child from crying. Chronic subdurals arising from birth trauma are very unlikely. Retinal haemorrhages due to birth trauma resolve within a few days. Children who suffer tears and bleeds to the brain substance will have long term developmental, neurological, intellectual and psychiatric difficulties.

Burns and scalds   About 10% of those who present with NAI have burns and about 10% of those who present with burns are due to abuse. While most physical abuse occurs under 2 years of age, deliberate burns and scalds peak in the third year. Improbable accidents do sometimes occur and unusual burns in those with pain insensitivity such as those with autism, intellectual disability and other neurological disorders need special care in their evaluation. Severe warning signs include burns on the face, the back of the hands, buttocks, legs, feet, perineum and genitalia, characterised by discrete shapes suggestive of cigarette burns, a clear "tide" mark on feet, ankles or wrists, and grid marks from fires and metal grills.

Accidental burns and scalds are more likely to affect face, shoulders, upper arms, and trunks. Accidental scalding from hot baths usually leaves irregular splash marks and burns to the hand are usually to the palm.

Investigations

These should include:

- Medical photography of bruises
- Coagulation studies to exclude a bleeding disorder
- Skeletal survey and nuclear bone scan
- CT or MRI of head where head injury has occurred or is suspected
- Ophthalmological examination in head injury
- Liver function tests and abdominal CT or MRI where abdominal injury is suspected. Note that persistent tachycardia in a child under 5 who is semicomatosed should raise the possibility of occult bleeding.

Management

All examinations and procedures should be conducted thoroughly and professionally, with all conclusions carefully and clearly documented. Emergency treatment should be provided as necessary regardless of the need to gather evidence. The local child protection team should be involved at the earliest opportunity by notifying the view that the child is at risk and stating the grounds for concern. If parents attempt or threaten to remove a child who is in imminent danger of abuse or who requires emergency treatment, the police and social services should be notified immediately. No attempt should be made personally to remove the child from the parents. A case conference of all those involved in the care of the child should be convened as soon as possible. When all this has been done the parents should be informed of the concerns and actions and the underlying reasons. This should only be carried out where it can be done safely.

For more specific measures see under the management of sexual abuse below, the principles of which are very similar.

Prognosis

For most children who are chronically abused there is a lifelong legacy. However, it must also be emphasised that most children who are abused do not become abusers even though most people who abuse have been abused. Those who have central nervous system damage carry the greatest burden of handicap with increased learning difficulties, psychiatric difficulty, and in some cases physical handicap such as paresis. Those most likely to be abusive themselves include those chronically abused who had parents with sadistic and highly developed rationales for abuse.

Sexual abuse

The definition of sexual abuse is the involvement of children in the sexual behaviour of adults. Severity is usually based on the degree of intrusion, threat, coercion, injury, chronicity, and long term sequelae. While the abuser is usually male and a member of the child's household, this is not exclusively so. Frequently, abused male children engage in sexually abusive acts of younger children. Sexual abuse may occur in any socioeconomic level in society but is more often reported in the poor. Types of sexual abuse include exposure to indecent acts, genital fondling, being forced or encouraged to masturbate an adult, through to various degrees of penetration.

Risk factors

These include:

- Previous history of sexual abuse in the family
- New male cohabitee in an already troubled household
- Male in household with history of sexual offences
- Sexual rejection of father by mother
- Recent sexual development of children reaching menarche.

Presenting features

Incidental disclosure

Common factors that work against disclosure include threats to the child, their siblings, their mother, friends, the family income, shame, and even the threat of the perpetrator going to gaol. Those engaged in repetitive paedophile behaviour are often skilled in identifying and exploiting the child's greatest fears. However, occasionally children, especially preschool children, are unaware that other children do not experience what they have experienced, and volunteer it by way of information.

Related medical presentations

Urinary tract infection, red buttocks, perineal soreness, anal bleeding, vaginal discharge and associated bruising may all provide the first clue of abuse. Sexually transmitted disease and pregnancy need to be considered in even quite young teenagers. Children who are homeless and engaged in prostitution for survival may present with sexually transmitted diseases at any age.

Non-specific psychiatric presentation

Children who have become socially withdrawn, failing at school against expectations with concentration difficulties, self-injurious behaviour and unexplained suicide attempts may all be exhibiting the outward expression of entrapment, threat, and abuse. More generally, any condition such as depression, anxiety, conversion disorder and anorexia may be triggered by abuse. Adolescent onset encopresis and enuresis in girls is especially worrying, particularly when they occur by day as well as night. Children who run away from home or are reluctant to leave hospital present particular concern.

Related psychiatric presentation

Sexualised behaviour may occur in those who are or have been sexually abused. It may also occur in those previously exposed to sexually explicit situations or material when anxious or excited. It may occur in children who have found reprieve from abusive situations as a result of adults realising the significance of their behaviour. These children may then reinvoke the behaviour almost unwittingly when anxious, frustrated, or angry. This may lead to confusion for carers and agencies responsible to supervise care. Another source of confusion may be in the thought content of those with obsessive compulsive disorder and those with psychoses. These may be bizarre and distressing to the young person and their families. Unless there is clear evidence of current abuse the clinician is wise to treat the primary condition first before attempting to evoke child protection investigation or legislation. Psychosis and obsessive compulsive disorder are not evidence per se of abuse even if the content of thought is explicitly sexual. Rarely psychogenic vomiting may arise in those involved in coercive oral sex.

Management

Reassure these children that you:

- Think it was a good thing to tell you of their abuse.
- Believe them and that you have taken what they have said seriously.

- Will do your utmost to prevent it happening again.
- Do not believe it is their fault and that they will not be punished by grown ups outside the family. Tell them that even grown ups we love do bad things sometimes.
- Know other children who had this happen to them who are now safe and well and happy.
- Will need to tell some people in order to keep them safe.

Take care to:

- Remain calm and relax the child.
- Listen carefully, and avoid leading and very specific questions early in the interview. Specific questions may be needed as the interview proceeds.
- Keep the parents, especially if one is the likely offender, onside but out of the interview.
- Have a colleague present to concentrate on documentation.
- Avoid confronting the likely offender.
- Eliminate multiple assessments.
- Prevent inexperienced people performing physical examinations or examinations under duress.
- Keep all professionals involved informed by regular updates by correspondence and case conferences.

Essential procedure

1. If there is a threat to life, such as haemorrhage, this must be dealt with first.
2. Document carefully.
3. Contact child protection specialists promptly.
4. Notify the social services, even if there is insufficient evidence but sufficient concern for the safety and welfare of the child.
5. A written notification should follow a verbal notification within 24 hours.
6. Physical examination with photography, examination with or without anaesthesia, colposcopy and microorganism culture is usually conducted by paediatric experts up to a week after the alleged abuse. Police are usually involved by this stage.

Emotional abuse

Definition

Habitual criticism, ridicule, humiliation, harassment, rejection or threat (verbal and non-verbal) or exposure to others undergoing this and other forms of abuse constitute emotional abuse. Emotional abuse and neglect commonly occur together. While there is much overlap, emotional abuse generally has greatest impact on behaviour and emotion and neglect has the greatest impact on development and capacity to form and sustain relationships.

Presentations

- Emotional flattening, social withdrawal and "looking away" behaviour in infants.
- Whining, miserable infants who cling to critical and unaffectionate parents.
- The still, passive toddler or young child who sits in "frozen watchfulness". In extreme cases this may present as mutism.
- Limited attention span, overactivity sometimes with marked anxiety.
- Indiscriminately friendly behaviour often craving adult approval and physical contact.
- Any form of psychiatric disorder but especially disruptive disorders.
- Learning difficulties abound in all who are relentlessly criticised and especially when this is combined with failure to help with schoolwork.
- Lowered self-esteem often leading to repetitive thoughts of suicide and preoccupation with death.
- Marked difficulties in peer relationships.
- Aggression, especially in boys and when emotional abuse is accompanied by physical abuse.

Management

- Indicate from the beginning a clear regard for these children and their welfare even where they are not particularly likeable. Be clear, however, that you are not nor can be their parent.

- Arrange whatever practical short term needs are required.
- Emphasise their strengths.
- Seek to minimise the total number of hours' exposure to the emotional abusive environment; for example extending preschool hours or arranging for afterschool care. These are important where removal from the emotional abuse has not been possible and therapeutic input is thought unlikely to be helpful or accepted.
- Case conferences including the school and other agencies to reduce secondary abuse by peers and unhelpful responses from teachers.
- Identifying important adults who might have a mentor role in the child's life, particularly in developing competencies that might promote resilience.

Neglect

Neglect is the failure to protect and provide for the child.

Presentations

- Infants who fail to thrive with their familes but thrive away from them.
- The infected infant or child with uncared for multiple minor skin infections such as impetigo or scabies.
- Severe and chronic nappy rash or excoriation due to failure to change nappies.
- Generalised developmental delay. In severe cases this may involve delay in speech, motor skills, and social development and responsiveness. It may involve short stature, microcephaly, and failure to develop urinary and faecal continence.
- Attachment disorders including anxious, avoidant, disorganised and reactive (largely failed) attachment pictures.
- The unkempt, dirty, child with very poor hygiene.
- Limited attention span, overactivity, social and emotional immaturity, and indiscriminate friendliness to strangers.

- Poor self-esteem.
- Aggressive, impulsive and antisocial behaviour, especially in the teenage years.
- Self-stimulating infants who may engage in rocking, head banging, and biting themselves. Older children may have "touch hunger" in which they seek physical closeness.
- Adolescents with self-injurious behaviour, poor coping skills, and who are sexually promiscuous.

Management

- Do what can be done for immediate problems and difficulties.
- Do thorough developmental assessments.
- Be aware of the likelihood of other forms of abuse.
- Try to reduce the total hours of exposure to neglectful environments.
- Try to increase exposure to sensory stimulation, social involvement, and healthy parenting.
- Inform by way of case conference, and where neglect is severe or persistent consider alternative care arrangements.

Conclusion

Neglect can be as damaging as any other form of abuse and can affect any aspect of the child's development and functioning. The possibility of reversing some of these impacts may diminish markedly after the age of 8 and even earlier with regard to language development.

Fabricated or induced illness by carer

Introduction

Fabricated or induced illness by carer is a syndrome in which a carer, more often the mother, falsifies physical or psychological illness in the child. The carer will then seek medical assessment and care, denying any knowledge as to the aetiology. The child may be subjected to multiple investigations and treatments, including surgery, despite repeated negative findings.

Illness may be falsified by either producing symptoms in the child by suffocation, injecting toxic substances, poisoning and bleeding, and/or illness is simulated with the mother presenting with factitious symptoms in her child. Simulated illness can be defined as illness falsified by the mother but not necessarily presenting with physical signs. Induced illness is where the mother inflicts illness on the child by directly causing harm to the child, for example by infecting a joint or contaminating a central line.

Thus fabricated or induced illness by carer is actually made up of a range of different situations:

- Provision of a false history and fabrication of symptoms
- Induction of physical symptoms and signs
- Interference with the treatment of an existing condition
- Failure to adequately nourish.

Poisoning

The perpetrator may use her own medications, common table salt, over the counter preparations, illicit drugs, and occasionally corrosives or more traditional poisons. Vomiting, diarrhoea, seizures, apnoea, hyperventilation, drowsiness and stupor, hallucinations, ulcerated mouth and very unusual blood profiles may all occur.

Suffocation

Mostly found in infancy but may occur during the first few years of life. The clinician should be suspicious if there are:

- Inexplicable episodes of apnoea
- Other unexplained conditions
- Other children who have been ill or died in unusual or unexplained circumstances
- Associated features of suffocation such as little burst blood vessels on the face, eyelids and inside the mouth, together with a generalised swelling of the face

- No episodes when the child is apart from the mother or suspected perpetrator.

The most common presentations include:

- Apparent bleeding from various sites—haematemesis, haematuria, haemoptysis, melaena, and epistaxis
- Central nervous system presentations—seizures, altered consciousness, ataxia, and nystagmus
- Respiratory involvement—apnoea from smothering
- Cardiac involvement—cyanosis, bradycardia, tachycardia, and hyperventilation
- Gastrointestinal involvement—diarrhoea, vomiting, abdominal pain, and anorexia
- Non-specific symptoms—fever, rash, arthralgia, septic arthritis, skin infections, immunodeficiency, glycosuria, and poisoning.

General Comments

Other forms of abuse may coexist.

It is important to check the history with collateral information. For example if the child has allegedly had a seizure in the presence of others; these observers should be interviewed. Finally it is important to review all consultations that the patient has had with other specialists, even if this involves wading through large files.

In over 70% of those with fabricated or induced illness by carer, illness will be produced and/or simulated within the hospital. There is also, not unusually, a past or current history of another family member similarly afflicted. The majority of perpetrators will do so in the hospital environment so this is a good place to confirm the diagnosis. There needs to be a planned strategy with all members of staff. A video camera may be necessary in extreme circumstances. Debate may focus on the ethics of entrapment rather than the safety of the child.

A further source of morbidity lies in the subsequent multiple investigations and procedures by medical staff. In other words, abnormal illness behaviour often elicits abnormal treatment behaviour. Almost all cases revolve around the quality of paediatric evidence. Often, mistakenly, paediatric staff have an expectation that psychiatric clinicians will provide the diagnostic information required. However, the essential evidence is paediatric history and symptoms without evidence or with evidence of production, simulation, or fabrication.

The most useful psychiatric information is usually the mother's personal medical history. The mother may be from a health related background such as nursing. Perpetrators tend to be people with good social skills and very persuasive and convincing. There is often a history of psychiatric disorder and the perpetrators often thrive in the hospital environment. However up to 20% do admit to the deception.

Demography

The incidence is unknown but it is possible that there are many undiagnosed cases. Boys and girls are affected equally, and it is most common in the early years, although cases have been reported of fabricated or induced illness by carer occurring in much older children.

Treatment

There is very little written about effective modes of treatment for fabricated or induced illness by carer. Recommendations include:

- Protect the child immediately and report suspected cases to social services, with the aim of holding a case conference at the earliest opportunity.
- Cases should be handled by a multidisciplinary protection team.
- The clinician's task is not to determine whether fabricated or induced illness by carer has occurred but whether the child is at substantial risk of deteriorating in the care of the parents or caregivers.
- When explaining the diagnosis to the family it is important to be supportive and not accusatory. The perpetrator may accuse medical staff of fabricating illness. Speak of your concerns and inform them that professional obligation requires social services involvement and protection for the child. It is advisable to organise a court hold on the child from the outset.

- Parental visits should be supervised by an experienced person at all times and there should be restrictions on parents bringing any food, drink or medication.
- Through the multidisciplinary team and case conferences, decisions must be made about the viability of the child ultimately returning to the perpetrating parent. Very careful consideration is required and the child's safety and well being must be foremost. Such decisions must not be rushed and if rehabilitation is to be attempted this must be within the context of the perpetrator accepting responsibility for the abuse and agreeing to very close supervision and support.

Prognosis

Up to 10% of victims of fabricated or induced illness by carer die and others suffer permanent disfigurement, impairment of function, or psychiatric disorder.

Conclusion

Although appalling to contemplate, if child maltreatment is not considered as a possible explanation for a child's ill health, then it will not be recognised. The busy clinician needs to be aware of all the possible presentations. Careful assessment is essential, as is involvement of a multidisciplinary team and social services. Urgent decisions must be made about the most suitable arrangements for the child's health, safety, and well being.

Further reading

Jones D. *Interviewing children who have been sexually abused*, 4th edn. London: Royal College of Psychiatrists/Gaskell Press, 1992.

Skuse D, Bentovim A. Physical and emotional maltreatment. In: Rutter M, Taylor E, Hersov L, eds. *Child and adolescent psychiatry: modern approaches*, 3rd edn. Oxford: Blackwell Science, 1994: chapter 13.

Williams DT. Somatoform disorders, factitious disorders and malingering. In: Narhpitz JD, ed. *Handbook of child and adolescent psychiatry. Vol 2. The grade school child: development and syndromes*. New York: Wiley, 1997:563–78.

19: The bereaved child

Introduction

Loss of any kind will have a profound effect on a child and most will experience it in one form or another by the time they reach adulthood. This chapter focuses specifically on the loss of the mother or father. The loss of grandparents, siblings, friends, pets, other loved ones and parental divorce can also have profound effects on the child. The bereavement process and its management is likely to be very similar.

Approximately 1 in 25 children in developed countries will suffer from the loss of a parent before 18 years of age, and the figure will be much higher in less prosperous and strife-ridden societies. The experience of such a loss for a child will depend on a number of factors. These include the developmental stage of the child, the quality of the relationship lost, the context of the death, and the ways in which the remaining members of the family are coping. Each of these factors will be considered in turn, followed by the management of grief generally.

Definition

Bereavement is the loss of a loved one through death. *Grief* is the intense emotional disturbance experienced following the loss, and *mourning* is the psychological process triggered by the loss.

Normal developmental concepts

In general in the younger age group the response to loss will be fundamentally one of separation. In the preschool years most children are unable to understand the permanency of death. Later they are able to understand the permanency. The mourning process will depend on the child's ability to retain a mental image of, and a range of emotional associations with, the lost person. This will, in turn, depend on the developmental level of the child and the nature of the relationship with those who are continuing to care for the child.

First two years

From the first few weeks babies are able to discriminate between their own mother and other women. Stranger anxiety emerges around 8 months with an insistence of at least visual contact with a parent, peaking at 18 months. In the first 6 months the concept of another person's permanence is not established and the inability of infants to hold a clear picture of the absent person will affect the ways in which they respond. This may protect the child from the emotional impact of separation because attachment has not yet occurred. From the end of the first year the child will be increasingly able to hold a representational image of an absent mother, conceptualising her as a separate entity, seeking her out when she is absent. The relationship will depend on the fit between mother and child, the child's temperament, and the mother's accommodation to it. As the child's attachment grows the vulnerability to bereavement grows.

Some have taken the young infant's inability to conceptualise constancy as evidence that separation of any sort may equate to death in this age group. It is true that children become very distressed and that this distress has features analogous to grief. However, there is no evidence that infancy is a process of continuous mourning. The extent of the effect of bereavement on the infant will depend on how abrupt and prolonged are the arrest of the provision of the baby's needs and on how long it takes for an alternative carer to take over the maternal role.

Toddlers too have difficulty understanding the finality of death, but will respond to the absence of their mother by searching for her. This may lead to the child becoming frightened when there is no response. The preparation prior to the death and the way the rest of the family copes in terms of accepting the new situation will influence the infant. Therefore in this age group the response will in essence be one of separation with clinging, crying, a need for attachment figures to always be in sight, with possible disturbances of sleeping, eating, and sometimes withdrawal. Bereavement in toddlers is especially hard. They are old enough to know what is happening but not old enough to make sense of it. Grief is often manifest in heedless overactivity or a clinging, wordless, withdrawn reduction in activity. The process of mourning is fitful, seemingly superficial, and sandwiched in between normal play and trivial interest in unrelated details. It is often missed because it is so often mingled with the day to day activities of the toddler. There is an increased risk of depression and antisocial behaviour associated with those who have lost a parent in the early years.

Two to five years

As children approach their third year, they begin to have a picture of the past and anticipate future events. Separations are followed by an expectation of reunion. As with all age groups, recently acquired skills are likely to be lost at this time of stress. Children who were continent may become incontinent. Some children speak in a more regressed speech pattern, and others have escalation in attachment behaviours such as whining, clinging, and refusal to sleep in their own beds. They may become defiant and aggressive, losing recently gained self-control skills. By way of contrast, they may also try to help by being good as a means of "making things better". In this age group it would not be unusual for a need for the story of the loss to be repeated many times with an emphasis on what happened, the sequence of events, and a very simplified explanation of causes.

When a child has previously had a concept of death from stories read or pets dying it is easier for them to understand the death of someone loved. Children may harbour fears that if they go to sleep or become sick they may die. Further losses of even minor things such as toys or pets may result in grief associated with the main loss and therefore result in what seems to be an inappropriate overreaction. Such opportunities should be taken to discuss the main loss and upset.

The child may become angry with either the dead or surviving people, particularly if that person has withdrawn within his own grief. Alternatively, children may withdraw, which may be misinterpreted as "coping", or search persistently, yearning for the dead person. Tearfulness is common, as is sleep, appetite, bowel and bladder disturbances, and general anxiety. The mourning process can continue over a period of months to years. Part of this process may involve intensification of attachments with people of a similar age and gender as the dead person. It is common for children to grieve in a fragmentary, frequently interrupted and poorly articulated manner. Children playing at funerals, seemingly unaware of the gravity of the situation typify this.

Five to eight years

Despite parental relationships being of prime importance, children in this age group can become attached to other adults such as teachers. They undergo moral and cognitive development, with a capacity for guilt about the past and anxiety about the future. An ability to contain and control feelings also begins.

By the age of 5 the development of the concept of death has commenced and by 8 years children have an understanding similar to adults. Nonetheless the death may be seen as a result of the child's actions and wishes. In this age group denial of the loss may be very prominent with an appearance of carrying on as normal even though the child's inner world may be significantly affected. Subsequently, the child's need to grieve may be ignored. Attempts may be made to keep the relationship with the lost person within their imagination. If substitute care is available and adequate, with family continuity, the mourning process will be generally settling at the end of a year.

When ambivalence existed in relation to the dead parent, care was inadequate subsequent to the death, the child was not informed supportively, or the losses were multiple, then there may be a more protracted and pathological course. Bereaved children may also be anxious about losing the other parent, as well as sensitive to the grief reaction of the remaining parent. The child may identify with loved and hated aspects of the dead person, including sometimes identifying with the parent's illness.

Eight to twelve years

Issues discussed earlier also apply to this age group. Relationships with friends become more important but still do not weigh as heavily as familial ties. As puberty begins the child may start to identify more with one parent and become more distant from the other. This will alter the response to the death of that parent. Not only have children of this age an understanding of death that is similar to that of adults but also a comprehension of their own mortality and the fears that accompany it. Consequently the death of another heralds the possibility that the child too may die. Now that the child can conceptualise a future, so with death the child also feels the sadness that comes with the knowledge of the anticipated loss for the future.

As do adults, children of this age react to death with shock, denial, anxiety, distress, tearfulness, and fear. Though now less dependent on parents than younger children, they may feel helpless and subsequently regress. Overtly, they may appear to be managing, but this may be just a response to what they feel is expected of them. Anger and irritability may surface against the surviving parent, younger siblings, or friends.

In those children who fail to resolve the loss and suppress the yearning, an idealised fantasy relationship with the dead person may form. It is therefore important that the child's need for mourning, with yearning, hopelessness and sadness, be supported. The child may withdraw, show some deterioration in schoolwork, or adopt behaviour associated with the lost person. Alternatively, they may act in a more mature manner and display compulsive care giving towards the surviving adult and siblings, giving the care desired for themselves.

Loss in adolescence

Important relationships for adolescents include both family and friends. However, generally the biggest loss an adolescent can have, particularly in the early teens, is the death of a parent. As with the other age groups the initial response is that of shock, numbness and disbelief, followed by yearning and longing for the dead person. Adolescents may try to resist overt yearning by denial. Anger is also common, fuelled by feelings of desertion, thoughts of future deprivation, resentment, loss of control, and a sense of unfairness. Depression, feelings of emptiness and somatisation are common responses. The adolescent mourning may be suppressed due to uncertainty of how others would react, worries about losing emotional control, concerns about looking abnormal, and sensitivity to peer evaluation. They are typically unsure about what is normal and so are hesitant about responding spontaneously. Adolescents find both friends, family and significant others helpful in coping, with girls talking more freely than boys. When possible preparation through open discussion prior to the death is also helpful.

The quality of the relationship lost

The degree and quality of the relationship and attachment to the lost person is of fundamental importance. A securely attached infant is likely to recover well from the loss, providing there is good quality alternative parenting and no major change to the socioeconomic standing of the family. By contrast, insecurely attached infants and anxious/avoidant infants may cope less well. However there is generally a strong tendency towards resilience and recovery in most children.

The context of the death

Expected versus unexpected loss

Expected loss occurs when the child is aware that the parent is dying and thus can prepare prior to the death. In sudden loss the death is unexpected. Others may have expected it, but perhaps, as a result of the developmental stage of the child, the child is unable to anticipate the loss. Children who are involved and informed when a loved one is terminally ill are able to start to work through the grief process in advance. The child may be able to say goodbye and discussion can begin about the loss.

In sudden loss there is no time for preparation or explanation. The remaining adults will also find the situation difficult to cope with and subsequently hard to explain. In addition, the child may have witnessed the death and so be suffering not only from grief but also the after effects of trauma.

Suicide

The child who loses a parent through suicide has specific additional problems. There may be shame and stigmatisation. The child may not be told of the nature of the death but still have suspicions. Some may even have witnessed the act or have discovered the body. Guilt, shame and resentment may complicate the mourning. Such bereavements are harder to recover from and depression is common.

Other losses

The death of a grandparent or sibling will still result in the same grief but to a lesser intensity. The death of a sibling will be particularly hard if there is a small age gap or if the sibling is a twin. The degree of mourning will once again depend on the nature of the relationship. When a sibling dies the parents may react by overprotection of the other children, treating a remaining child as a replacement for the dead child, or idealising the dead child with the remaining children feeling as if they fall short of their parents' expectations.

Styles of grieving

There are many pathological forms of grieving.

Silent grief

In some families the death is never discussed. The children are kept in the dark when a family member is terminally ill. They will nonetheless sense that something dreadful is happening but feel unable to talk about it. They may be told nothing at the time of death or that the person has gone away or gone to heaven. The secrecy surrounding the death may make them feel uncomfortable in asking questions. Most of all there is a lack of freedom to mourn and so grief may remain unresolved.

Guilty grief

Some families have a need to find fault. This is especially so if, prior to the death, the family used guilt as a tool to enforce discipline together with high expectations and control of the children. Generally this is matched with unresolved guilt in the parents, which becomes misplaced onto others. A person is sought to blame for the death and guilt is the dominant reaction to the death. In addition, if these families find it hard to adapt to change, the challenge of finding new roles for each member of the family subsequent to the bereavement will be difficult. The predominant theme of guilt may hinder adaptation to loss and therefore to mourning. Even when families do everything appropriately, children may still feel guilt.

A private and postponed grief

Some families' relationships are more reserved. The parents may have previously experienced traumatic separation and losses. When someone dies it would be considered too distressing to allow expression of intense emotions related to grief for fear of opening up old wounds. The mourning is noted and placed "on the back burner", postponed, with an outward appearance of coping well. Children may be confused by intense personal feelings compared to the apparent lack of overt suffering in their parents and learn to dampen their own emotions.

A fragile grief

In families with few financial and psychological resources the death may result in marked disruptions in daily life. Frequently, prior to the loss, these vulnerable family members have suffered from psychiatric disorders, tenuous adjustment, sickness, and loss. They normally have few supports outside the family other than from professional agencies. The family runs the risk of disintegrating and the children may be placed into care. Their losses are therefore multiple, including the family unit, the home as well as the deceased relative.

An ordinary grief

However in those families who are open and share emotions, where most relationships are valued and where the positive emotions can be tolerated along with the negative, healthy mourning can occur. Prior to the loss these children are much more likely to have learned that angry and sad feelings will be tolerated, and responded to with comfort. The loss is very painful for all but the resources are in place for the family to grieve healthily. The family adapt for the most part. Any conflicts that were present at the time of death are usually resolved over time because of the family's strength and resilience. The child, though hurting, is able to be comforted and cared for and grief is expressed.

There are of course many exceptions to this general picture. For example children from appalling backgrounds may cope well and children from the most open and communicative of families may cope poorly. Such individual differences pervade child psychiatry. However in general the freedom to grieve, free of guilt, with support and love usually leads to satisfactory resolution.

The needs of the bereaved child

Each child will have a different combination of needs depending on their developmental age and situation. The most common of these are described below.

Reassurance

Children need to be reassured verbally and non-verbally that they are still loved and valued, and that further disasters will not ensue, and that they are not responsible for the death. It is both reassuring and slightly surprising for young children to find out that they are not so powerful as to have caused another person to have died, and they are safe from any retribution. These seemingly unlikely thoughts are not at all uncommon. They are not pathological and their acceptance and understanding can be very reassuring.

Stability and normality

A stable environment is important and as soon as possible normal day to day activities such as schooling should be resumed. Normal discipline is still needed for inappropriate behaviour to provide structure and security, while recognising that greater tolerance is needed.

Questions and answers

Common questions, based on age and level of maturity, include "why did mummy die", "was it because I was naughty", "where has mummy gone", "will her body get wet in the cemetery", "will she be in pain when she is cremated", "what is it like in heaven", or "can she see me".

Answers should be as clear, honest, factual and age appropriate as possible. Death should not be likened to sleep, for this may create a fear of sleep. By answering questions openly and sympathetically we are acknowledging and accepting the child's grief as well as helping them to cope.

Opportunity to say goodbye

If there is an opportunity to say goodbye before death this should be taken. Otherwise goodbyes can be said at the funeral or by a letter or drawings. Children may well want to put some flowers, a letter, a photograph or gift in the coffin, and this should be very much supported. It is useful to describe beforehand what will happen at a funeral.

Physical contact

Much cuddling and comforting is usually wanted and needed during the grieving period and this should be liberally available, but not of course imposed.

Support of bereaved children

The person best placed to support a bereaved child is the remaining parent. The clinician's responsibility is to advise and support the carer in this task. Carers are themselves experiencing intense grief and may well need support in this task. Memory boxes or scrapbooks can be used to contain special memorabilia of the lost person. Should children wish it is perfectly appropriate for them to talk to others outside the family, such as a valued friend, the family doctor, or a member of the religious group to which they belong. Bereavement groups may be helpful.

Psychiatric disorders complicating bereavement

It is important to differentiate the normal bereavement process with its associated depressive and anxiety symptoms from a psychiatric disorder. Those to be considered include depression (see chapter 6), separation anxiety (see chapter 3), and post-traumatic stress disorder (see chapter 4).

Long term effects of childhood bereavement

There is limited information on the long term effects of bereavement. Later psychiatric disorder appears to be quite common. Poor outcome is more likely when the surviving parent is unable to provide good parenting or when the bereaved child has had a poor relationship with either parent, unless the bereavement serves to free a child from an aversive or abusive situation. Men who have been bereaved in childhood have a higher incidence than expected of criminal offences, major medical illness, and emotional distress. It is surprising how often children adjust well to bereavement.

Further reading

Breier A, Kelsoe JR, Kirwin PD, Beller SA, Wolkowitz OM, Pickar D. Early parental loss and development of adult psychopathology. *Archives of General Psychiatry* 1988;**45**:987–93.

Furman E. Bereavement of the grade school child. In: Noshpitz JP, ed. *Handbook of child and adolescent psychiatry*. Vol 2. *The grade school child: development and syndromes*. New York: Wiley, 1997: chapter 23.

Guthrie J, Weller R, Weller E. Childhood bereavement. In: Noshpitz JP, ed. *Handbook of child and adolescent psychiatry*. Vol 4. *Varieties of development*. New York: Wiley, 1997:32–8.

Hallam B, Vine P. Expected and unexpected loss. In: Lindsay B, Elsegood J, eds. *Working with children in grief and loss*. London: Baillière Tindall, 1996:56–72.

Raphael B. *The anatomy of bereavement. A handbook for the caring profession*. London: Hutchinson, 1984.

20: The dying child

Introduction

The death of a child in industrialised society is relatively rare, though sadly far more common in developing countries. For those affected the impact is devastating. In helping people through the death of a child there is little known about effective interventions. As a result the clinician must draw heavily upon skills of empathy and compassion.

Epidemiology

In the UK, approximately 1% of births ends in stillbirth with a further 1% dying in the first 4 weeks of life. For the statistics thereafter see Table 20.1.

Developmental issues

Children understand very little of the permanency of death before 5 or 6 years (see chapter 19). Greater understanding of death usually occurs if the child has lost a pet or relative.

Clinical issues

The child's perspective

This varies with age and maturity. The terminally ill child is likely to fear pain and separation as well as death itself. Older children will, in addition, sense parental anxieties and distress. This may be aggravated by failure to discuss what is happening. Children's sense of loss of control of their lives may be expressed in their attempts to regain control by testing behaviour. Adolescents who normally fight for increasing autonomy may

Table 20.1 Common causes of death in childhood

Age	Approximate death rate per 10 000	Commonest causes
4 weeks to 1 year	7	Congenital anomalies
1–5 years	7	Accidents and congenitial anomalies
5–15 years	3	Accidents and malignancy

find the loss of control all the more profound. In addition, adolescents who already have to cope with a changing body will also have the additional effects of the illness or treatment, such as alopecia and weight loss, at a time when peer approval is so important. Children and adolescents may feel anger and resentment at being ill and express it towards their parents.

The parent's perspective

The parents of children with chronic and terminal illness will experience grief on a number of different occasions along the path of the illness. First they will feel the loss of the child's future, "anticipatory mourning", further distress as the illness progresses, and "terminal grief" at the time of death. At each stage they are likely to experience the natural phases of grief, shock, denial, depression, anger, and hopefully then adaptation. Each phase can last for days or weeks and sometimes months.

Parents may feel unable to protect their child, resulting in increased care giving behaviour, or actually be so distressed that they cannot provide adequate parenting. Pre-existing problems, such as marital disharmony or alcohol abuse, may intensify. Alternatively the adversity to be faced may elicit great strength and resilience.

Management

This must give consideration not only to the sick child but also to the whole family. In assessing the families of dying children it is important to elucidate what the child knows and understands about the illness, what concerns exist, what supports are in place, and what future stresses may occur. What the child knows and understands may be quite different to what the child has been told, so it is best not to assume information is known. It is important to facilitate an atmosphere in which the child feels nothing is unspeakable, including death. However it is also necessary to acknowledge that different members of the family will have different needs and different ways of coping. Parents may fear that the news will be too much for their child to handle. With help and support parents can often be persuaded that their child needs to be able to talk about dying. To avoid doing so will create an emotional distance between them and their child when support is what is most needed. A rule of thumb is that the older the child is the more appropriate it is to talk about their death.

The dying child may experience depression, anger, and anxiety. When these interfere with the quality of life or care, or these emotions are overwhelming, it may be necessary to prescribe short term anxiolytics and antidepressants (see chapter 25).

The child is likely to spend time both in and out of hospital. Hospitalisation may intensify separation issues for the child and family. Some admissions, may correctly or otherwise, be viewed by the child, as the end drawing closer. This makes it all the more important to be as open as possible with the terminally ill child. The family needs to feel supported, informed, and understood. Parents may be helped, by feeling involved with their child's care, in particular when the child is young, as well as sleeping in the same room. Dying children should be supported in any wish to maintain a social network through telephone calls, letters, and visits. Every effort must be made to help the patient and family to feel more in control, such as allowing both to be involved in as many of the decision making processes as possible. Choices can be given about options in hospital daily life, and how they would like to make the hospital room more personal. Children will generally worry about pain and they need to feel reassured that this will be well managed. Parents and children can be introduced to others in similar situations, either in formal groups, or informally.

If the child is still undergoing painful or uncomfortable procedures and treatments, it is important to explain as clearly as possible what is happening. This enables the child to feel some sense of control. Using toys and dolls in advance to perform mock procedures may help. During the procedure parental presence and comforting, and distraction such as using visual images and blowing bubbles, can help. Deep muscle relaxation and hypnosis can help the older child.

In the final stages even more effort should be made to ensure that the child's and family's wishes and needs are being given every consideration.

Management of the grieving parent

The loss of a child produces the greatest intensity of bereavement. The family may desire some time to be alone with their child and this should be provided. Parents may blame themselves for no good reason. They need to be reassured of the limits of what they could have done. The parents should be given an opportunity at a later date to ask all the questions they need answered when initially none may come to mind.

Sudden deaths are frequently the hardest to manage. This is made worse when there were possible actions that parents could have taken to prevent the death. They are usually not familiar with the hospital staff and follow up in the community is sometimes unsatisfactory. By contrast, for the child who had a protracted terminal course, relationships have been built in the hospital and the parents may receive more attention and concern.

All families should be offered bereavement counselling following their child's death, and the opportunity to remain in contact with the staff.

Talking about death

The following points may be helpful, whether such a conversation occurs when the parents are first being told about the inevitability of death, or immediately after the child's death:

- Maintain eye contact
- Quiet room with no interruptions
- Allow plenty of time
- Do not talk too quickly or too much
- Avoid medical jargon and keep the facts clear and simple
- Silence is alright
- Listen
- Support emotional expression by parents
- Ask what they would find helpful
- Respect the parents' reactions, whatever they might be
- Give the parents time on their own at the end in the room where the interview took place.
- Offer follow up

Conclusion

Helping the dying child is always a draining and emotionally demanding task. Helping the parents of the dying child requires a sensitivity that supports them without displacing their role as parents. Learning how to share bad news is an important skill, which requires patience, sensitivity, and openness. Uncertainty, pain, fear of separation and unforeseen complications may all interfere with trust or lead to deeper trust. The clinician's ability to negotiate these difficulties will often determine the quality of life of children during their last days and the memories that their parents have.

Further reading

Koocher G, Gudas L. Death and dying. In: Noshpitz J, ed. *Handbook of child and adolescent psychiatry*. Vol 4. *Varieties of development*. New York: Wiley, 1997:76–88.

Selter L. The dying child. In: Jellinek M, Herzog D, eds. *Psychiatric aspects of general hospital paediatrics*. Chicago: Year Book Medical Publishers, 1990:272–7.

Section III
Treatment

21: Treatment overview

Introduction

This chapter tackles management with particular emphasis on the shift from assessment to treatment and from symptomatic relief to management of the underlying problems. There is also, woven into this approach, a steady progression from immediate to longer term management. The emphasis is on what is pragmatically useful to the clinician in helping the child and family rather than the pursuit of a supposed ideal approach to treatment. At each point the goal is to be as helpful as possible using an economy of clinical effort. Allied to this is the importance of adopting a comprehensive approach within the context of a therapeutic alliance.

We believe that clinicians should provide treatment from the moment of first contact. Thus assessment and treatment overlap. In chapter 2 we have considered assessment separately but it continues throughout the treatment process, as will be illustrated in this chapter.

With regard to management, all treatments have something to contribute while none at present provides all the answers. A comprehensive approach that includes psychological, family and medical factors is essential. In succeeding chapters we focus on the specifics of various therapeutic approaches and in earlier chapters we have referred to the specific treatments indicated for each condition. In this chapter we focus on the general principles.

Short-term management—what to do immediately

The presenting problems do not always appear connected to a particular organ system, nor necessarily fit into any recognised pattern. Rather they are the subjective reflection of distress or discomfort. Treatment therefore involves starting with attempts to relieve the immediate distress rather than searching for deeper underlying meaning. Thus in child psychiatry we might start with a child who:

Box 21.1 General principles of treatment

- Be as positive as possible with children and parents. They need and appreciate all the encouragement they can get
- Offer support and advice but don't take over from the parents. The main task is to help parents help their child
- Keep in mind the child and parent's perspectives simultaneously
- Avoid parental requests to be a friend or an authority to the child
- Help a child to be able to put forward his/her view in any assessment or treatment
- Beware of the belief that we can do what others have failed to achieve
- Always adopt a comprehensive approach, paying due attention to psychological, social and physical factors
- Different children and different problems need different treatments
- Whenever possible use treatments for which there is good evidence of effectiveness
- Don't avoid child protection issues

- Feels sad or anxious
- Is unwilling to go to school
- Has inconsistent medical signs without obvious disease basis
- Refuses to obey parental requests
- Comes from a distressed family with marital discord.

In time there will be a need to move from a medical formulation of disease to an understanding of possible psychological contributors. This may lead to a focus on family and particularly parenting issues, and even to an acknowledgement that all is not well with the marriage. The skilled clinician can often do this progressively, seamlessly, and in a minimum of time. Adopting a comprehensive approach rather than an "either physical or psychological" approach will reassure many parents that we as clinicians are not dismissing a potentially life-threatening condition as "all in their head". There are times, however, where no amount of diplomacy will avoid the fracturing effect upon the patient–clinician relationship. However there are some general principles of management applicable in any therapeutic context, regardless of the presenting problems, diagnosis, and treatments. These are summarised in Box 21.1.

Bearing in mind these general principles it is now appropriate to consider the specifics of symptomatic treatment.

The components and goals of symptomatic management

Each modality of treatment should have specific objectives and means for monitoring progress. The focus may equally be on the child and the family.

Symptomatic management of the family

Almost all negotiations about children involve working with their parents. Older teenagers may arrange independent agreements and younger children may be seen without parental permission when safety overrides consent. However, even in these situations there are benefits to be gained from involving the family unless it is clear that harm may be done.

Immediate support includes achieving a therapeutic alliance by ascertaining each person's views, acknowledging and accepting their validity. This allows for the necessary containing of anxiety, anger or other forms of distress. The clinician's task is then to offer an understanding of the problem as quickly as possible accompanied by information about the necessary treatment, the likely course and the probable outcome. Where possible, reassurance should be offered in relation to any parental fears of deterioration or chronicity.

Symptomatic management of the individual child

Pending the implementation of whatever specific psychological treatments may be indicated (for example addressing the child's thoughts and behaviour through cognitive behaviour therapy, the inner world of the child's relationships and feelings through psychodynamic psychotherapy, or the child's imagination as accessed through play and art therapies), other more immediate help may be indicated.

The busy clinician aims at safety first, symptomatic relief second, and then looking at the underlying sources of issues. These three Ss (safety, symptoms, sources) recur at every level of treatment.

Addressing potentially unstable medical conditions such as diabetes, epilepsy, starvation in anorexia nervosa and asthma may all have a beneficial effect on mental state. Taking trouble over self-inflicted lacerations, neglected hygiene, self-care, dental work and sexually transmitted diseases conveys a strong sense of concern.

The use of medication in child psychiatry is still largely symptom based. Many of the diagnostic categories are merely symptom clusters. The physiological distress of the child may require acute antianxiety drugs, sedation or even antipsychotic medication (see chapter 25) pending a more definitive diagnosis. These should always be considered as possible "first aid" prior to the implementation of a more comprehensive and indepth approach; equally, however, they should never be offered as an exclusive treatment.

Symptomatic monitoring

Pending a definitive formulation of the problems it is essential to check safety, distress, and the impact of treatment. The possibility of self-harm (see chapter 6), abuse (see chapter 18) or medical threat should always be considered.

Managing the psychosocial network

Stressors

Any attempt to help usually involves defining and, where possible, minimising the impact of stressors. Sometimes the stressors are particular people and relationships. In children who have attempted suicide, removal from the immediate family on a short term basis often dramatically reduces self-harming behaviour. Part of the clinical assessment is to determine those parts of the patient's interpersonal network that are supportive and those that are stressful.

Relief

An opportunity to gain relief from critical, conflictual, overprotective, violent, chaotic and generally adverse environments offers short term help while longer term social predicaments are being addressed.

Management

Priorities for the medium term

There is usually a subtle and seamless shift from the management of symptoms of distress to understanding and tackling the antecedents to the presentation. The predisposing, precipitating and perpetuating factors are slowly delineated. This is done through the collation of corroborative information and the consensus that arises from investigation. The wise clinician is trying to discern a predominant pattern in the clinical picture while nevertheless scanning for discrepancies to the common patterns. Interviewing the child and family provides a deeper understanding of the unique factors that have contributed to the child's condition. Standardised psychometric tests give an appreciation of how this child compares with other children. Educational assessment from the school or other specialist services enables the clinician to identify the role of specific and general learning difficulties in the presenting problem. Medical investigation by a thoughtful physician is always helpful, if not to diagnose, at least to reassure that there is no contributing medical disorder.

Slowly, all the possible causes are considered, a differential diagnosis is explored, and hopefully a definitive diagnosis made. Appropriate management of psychological, social and physical factors is now implemented.

With the transition from short to medium term management, there is also a shift to clarifying the definitive components of treatment. Identifying who is in charge, the time frame of treatment, the way in which different forms of treatment will be integrated and the nature and length of follow-up become the new priorities. Predicting which treatments are likely to work and which are not and when to stop treating are all difficult, but important, elements of this phase of treatment.

Long term management

In some situations chronicity occurs or is inevitable (for example a disease such as diabetes). In such cases a long term management plan is needed. This should consider how to ensure an adequate quality of life for the child, satisfactory adherence to treatment, increasing and age appropriate autonomy, transition to adult services and who is responsible for supervising treatment at each time point. Each of these issues is best tackled through open discussion with child and parents.

Adherence

Adherence with treatment of any kind is almost always partial. We should not be surprised at this or regard it as abnormal, but try to understand the factors that might reduce adherence and how best to enhance it. The more demanding, intrusive and longlasting the treatment regimen, the more likely that adherence will be inadequate. Creating an open atmosphere of frank discussion about what is unacceptable about different treatments is very helpful. Inviting constructive criticism of treatments can promote this while nevertheless retaining what may be helpful. It is helpful to encourage the child to consider the perceived disadvantages to complete adherence, for there will be many, for example treatment is boring, intrusive, interferes with social life, may have unpleasant side effects, etc. The acknowledgement of the validity of these views allied with a non-coercive approach is far more likely to yield a benefit than harassment, threats, "education", and coercion.

Transition to adult services should be planned well ahead, with careful consideration being given to the young person's needs. Ideally there should be a gradual transition with the possibility of shared care or at least occasional joint consultations.

Prognosis

Distress in the present can be relieved, endured or rendered intolerable by the prospects for the future. The following suggestions may prove helpful:

- Unless there is good reason to do otherwise be cautious about the short term and encouraging about the long term. It is rarely helpful to raise short-term expectations and to lower longer term expectations unless there is very good evidence to do so. Raising short term expectations of relief sets up for disappointment if they fail to be realised. Lowering longer term expectations induces despair and reduces motivation. There are times when this must be done but it needs to be based on some clear evidence. With most psychological disorders, lowering short term expectations and raising longer term expectations is the preferred strategy.
- *Manage uncertainty actively.* When improvement is experienced, warn of possible short term setbacks. When setbacks are experienced remind the family of improvements and past successes. If this is not done clinicians can end up following a clinical roller coaster of heightened expectations when improvement occurs and despair when setbacks occur. If it is clear that deterioration will occur this needs to be said definitely, supportively, and in plain English. Detailed descriptions of what will happen need to be left for nearer the time, unless the parents pre-empt this with their own fears. This is particularly true for palliative care when parents may differ in the timing of their need for information. Where there is uncertainty the elements of uncertainty need to be elaborated with what is known, what can be known, and what cannot be known. If investigations or other information are awaited, the implications of these findings for the future need to be discussed.
- *Emphasise the positive and the possibilities for action.* Identify positive prognostic features and emphasise those factors where the family and child can move things in a positive direction. Raise the issues of concern as a background factor so that the family will be clear that you are not merely putting a positive gloss on the facts. Do not minimise what they have been through or the difficulties

ahead. Do emphasise their resilience and how well they have managed to date. Prognosis looks better with sleep, time out, and an opportunity to adjust to new information.

- *Helping to understand the prognosis.* One helpful way to present information about the future is to illustrate the best case scenario, the worst case scenario, and the most likely case scenario. It is also important to distinguish the differences between the prognosis for the condition as a whole and the prognosis for the particular episode at the time. Sometimes the focus is on the prognosis for an especially troubling symptom or sign.

Ultimately, we must address the prognosis for the individual child. This individualised prognosis, rather than an epidemiological prognosis, involves anticipating possible complications, weighing assets against liabilities, and looking to prevent complications. It will involve a practical assessment of prognosis for lifestyle not only for the child but also for the rest of the family. Parents will also be proccupied with the prognosis for siblings and their children's children. In all of this the clinician is vigilantly monitored by the family as a prognostic barometer. It also becomes clear that the family responds to their child and the treatment process based on the clinician's portrayal of the future.

Now that we have examined how the treatment process should work, let us turn to what can go wrong.

Tips and traps

Responding to human need and distress has a long and noble tradition. It also seems self-evident that "something should and must be done". However, need and distress have their own difficulties and dangers for whoever decides to attempt to subdue, master, quell or assuage them. Any overview of treatment involves thinking about the problems of being helpful. There is an ever-present possibility of doing harm, making things worse, sinking in the struggles of others, and expanding the maelstrom of troubled hearts and minds.

When people are distressed, others who are helping may also be overwhelmed. However, it is important to be sure that we are capable of helping and are not moving too far from our previous experience base. Of course, we must get new experience and push ourselves beyond our "comfort zone". But this ought to be done steadily, thoughtfully and with opportunity to build progressively on previous experience. It helps if we can do this with another more experienced colleague, but sometimes this is not possible. Sometimes we have no one to support us and no one to whom to refer. It is imperative in this situation to gain links of support via telephone, out-of-town training, and very clearly defined treatment goals with the patient.

There are a number of potential pitfalls:

- Treating beyond or without consent.
- Trying to cure the incurable.
- Trying to manage the unmanageable.
- Criticising critical parents.
- Using favourite treatments rather than the ones the child and family need.
- Confusing our problems with those of our patients and their families.
- Failing to share our work with colleagues, keep up with current knowledge or obtain supervision.
- Blaming the patient for not getting better.
- Fighting with the child or family instead of fighting with the illness.
- Avoiding patients when things are not improving.
- Taking criticisms from children and their families personally.
- Failing to support the child's emerging need for autonomy.

Even the most experienced can be challenged by such scenarios. Good lines of support, supervision and administrative accountability are essential in helping us to avoid such pitfalls and to ensure the provision of excellent treatment.

Conclusion

Assessment and treatment overlap throughout clinical contact. Treatment should always be comprehensive, paying due attention to psychological, social and physical factors, within the context of a therapeutic alliance. It should be initiated early and should include symptomatic relief, as well as support and advice for the parents. There will be a gradual introduction of a more indepth approach where required. Attention should be paid to the differing perceptions, needs and attitudes of the children and their parents, with attention also being given to such issues as adherence and expectations of the future. When chronicity is an issue, adherence, quality of life and transition to adult care require special attention.

Further reading

Hubble MA, Duncan BL, Miller SD. *The heart and soul of change—what works in therapy.* Washington: American Psychological Association, 1999.

Nathan PEE, Goman JM. *A guide to treatments that work.* New York: Oxford University Press, 1998.

Seligman MEL. *What you can change and what you can't".* Sydney: Random House, 1999.

22: Parental and family treatment

Introduction

Childhood difficulties arise as a result of a wide range of circumstances (see chapter 1), by no means always to do with the family. However not infrequently family dysfunction does contribute to the emergence or maintenance of such problems. Once these have emerged the family is in the strongest position to help the child. In working with families the prime task is to help the family help the child. There are many different ways of helping families and many different schools of family counselling. However, all share the underlying assumption that many problems can arise from, be maintained by, or resolved within the family. Helping troubled children almost always involves working with and through their parents, and not infrequently may include other family members. This chapter offers an overview of such family-based treatments.

Family difficulties that may contribute to a child's problems

- *Lack of consistency.* Parental inability to work together consistently between each other or consistently over time (see below).
- *Parental conflicts.* An inability for parents to agree, make decisions and work together to solve problems, sometimes drawing the child(ren) in to the conflict (triangulation of the child).
- *Overwhelmed parents.* An inability for parents to respond to the stresses of daily living by failing to be organised themselves and failing to help the children to be organised.
- *Inflexible parenting.* Responding in too rigid a manner so that the proposed solutions to problems do not match the child's needs.

- *Enmeshed families.* Such closeness that individuals may have an impaired sense of their own feelings, autonomy, or even identity.
- *Absent or unsupportive parents.* Being so distant, disengaged or ineffectual that family members feel unsupported.
- *Alliances and coalitions.* Family members may have inappropriately close relationships, for example a parent and child (cross-generational), or even form a coalition against one or more other family members.
- *Emotionally out of tune.* One or both parents may be unable to recognise, accept or acknowledge the feelings of others (see below).
- *Faulty communication.* Many patterns are to be found, including: failure to listen or failure to respond; frequent interrupting; more than one person speaking at a time; one person dominating the conversations; poverty or excess of communication; discordant communication (when verbal and non-verbal communications do not correspond). None of these occurring occasionally is a problem, but frequent recurrence or persistence is likely to be problematic (see below).

Therapeutic alliance

Essential to any therapeutic endeavour is the creation of a therapeutic alliance—a key component of the therapeutic process (see also chapter 2). This involves creating a supportive relationship with the parents and family by conveying interest in and concern for their difficulties, respect for the efforts they have made, and commitment to helping them. It is maintained by empathy, attentive listening, positive regard, a non-judgemental attitude, and continuous emotional tracking of how each person feels.

Different types of help

Just as there are different surgical techniques for the same surgical problem and different clinical approaches for the same clinical condition, there are different ways of helping parents and families. Working with families involves many different levels of intervention—support, advice, parental counselling, and family therapy—each of which may be utilised in isolation or, more usually, combination, and at different times during the therapeutic process.

Support

There is nothing complicated about providing emotional support and this should be part of the repertoire of all clinicians. It does however require a degree of subtlety, in that it involves accessibility, attentive listening, acknowledgement, and acceptance of feelings. This is in itself supportive and helps the family to feel understood and validated in its concerns or distress, thus enhancing the potential for family coping.

Advice

This also is part of the clinical repertoire and usually involves offering carefully considered, specific and goal-directed advice. It has the advantage of giving the family some "concrete" ideas of how to proceed at a time when they are likely to be feeling demoralised and confused. In offering advice it is important that it is based upon a clear understanding of what precipitates or aggravates the problem, what has been tried so far, by whom, for how long, and with what results. Any advice offered thereafter should be acceptable to the responsible adult(s). There is little point in advising a particular approach if it is unacceptable.

Normally such advice is likely to be symptom orientated but may also focus on the way in which the parents deal with situations. For example, if a child is wetting the bed, symptom focused advice might include the suggestion that the child not drink fluids in the 4 hours before bedtime and be woken a couple of hours after falling asleep. This might be supplemented by advising the parents of the importance of agreeing an approach that is both consistent between each of them and consistent over time.

This emphasis on consistency forms a crucial component of work done with parents. All too often parents do not adopt a consistent approach, either by each adopting a different approach, or, although they may be consistent between each other they change their approach very frequently, with a subsequent and inevitable failure to resolve the difficulties. Usually whichever approach is adopted needs to be applied over several weeks. Therefore one of the most basic pieces of advice is that parents should work to find an approach to problem solving that is applied consistently between them and consistently over time.

Parental counselling

The essence of counselling is helping the parents find their own solutions and in so doing increasing their confidence and sense of effectiveness. Central to this way of working is exploration of the problems and their potential solutions. There needs to be exploration of:

- What seems to precipitate and what seems to aggravate the problems
- What has been tried with what results
- What would the parent(s) like to try next
- With what techniques or strategies do they feel comfortable and can offer mutual support in their application.

The aim is to enhance parental coping not by advising, instructing or prescribing, but by helping them to become more effective parents. The counsellor helps the parents set the agenda and find the solutions.

Family therapy

Working with various combinations of the family to explore and resolve precipitating and perpetuating factors. As with various other therapies there are many models of family therapy, and yet more are emerging. No one approach is likely to be superior to any other and most skilled therapists draw upon different styles and techniques, rather than being bound to one. The particular techniques used are likely to be based upon therapist preference and familiarity and what seems right for particular families. Different techniques may also be used at different times.

Some key principles underlie the practice of family therapy, and these include the following concepts:

- The family is a unit in itself as well as a group of individuals.
- Family structure is based on the different generations and their relationships.
- Individual behaviour, attitudes, communication patterns and emotionality is shaped by exposure to other family members and particularly parents.
- The symptoms that are causing concern may have a function of "helping" family stability or cohesiveness.
- Family relationships and behaviour change according to the stage of the life cycle.

These concepts inform the actual practice, some key elements of which are now discussed (see also chapter 2):

- Therapists should ensure that in each meeting they make direct and supportive contact with each family member. The aim is to ensure that each person feels included, respected and supported throughout the therapeutic process.
- Therapists should always attempt to devise a formulation which links the above features. This formulation will be constructed during the assessment but may alter as more information becomes available during the therapy. The formulation should be shared as much as possible with the family.
- The therapeutic goals should be based on the formulation and agreed between the members of the family and the therapist. There is little point in the therapist having one aim and the family another, or even different family members having different aims.
- Therapists should generally focus on and encourage direct interaction between family members rather than being the centre of activity themselves. Although in the initial stages of therapy the therapist is likely to be more active, in the later stages it is the family who should be doing most of the work. It is likely that if the therapist is talking a great deal or working very hard then the family is probably not working at change.

- Parental authority should always be acknowledged. It is all too easy for the parents to feel undermined by the therapist's expertise and competence. This is avoided by supporting the parents' role even when trying to help them change their parenting style.
- The family should be helped to seek solutions to their problems by exploring what hasn't worked and finding new strategies.
- There should be continuous evaluation of progress with the family.

The above principles should be universal to all styles of family therapy. However there are many different techniques in use and some of these are now discussed. They are not necessarily applied in all cases nor by all therapists, but judiciously and skilfully applied in the appropriate circumstances, they can be very useful.

In general the therapist should start with the presenting problem and exploring it in detail. When interviewing parents this means getting a description of the problem from each parent's point of view. When seeing the family as a whole it means seeing how every member of the family sees the problem and whether they see any other problems.

There are also differences between individuals as to which focus they prefer. Some people are very much focused on the present. Others prefer to understand why things might have occurred. Still other people are not nearly so worried about what the problem is or why it might have occurred but rather what they must do to correct the situation. Often a person of one style or focus has a partner of a different style or focus. The clinician must gently but persistently point out the different questions, concerns and expectations if disappointment or misunderstanding is to be avoided.

Specific techniques

Exploring the past

Many different types of therapy, including family therapy, examine the past to understand the present difficulties: "We are as we are because we were as we were". Attempts to understand the past may help to explain why the family is struggling now. One way of doing this is to construct a family tree (or genogram). Each person is represented with their names, ages, and personality characteristics. Illnesses, separations and other important family events can all be represented. The tree can go back as far as information is available. This can lead to a more detailed understanding of the development of the current problems, as much information can be gained from the way family members answer as from what they say. Such techniques may provide a greater understanding for the therapist and insight for the family. Whether insight is sufficient in itself for change is debatable, but it may certainly contribute.

"Here and now"

Some approaches to helping families emphasise working on what is happening in the "here and now". The therapist observes current interaction and relationship patterns and considers whether these are replications of the family's everyday patterns. For example, if mother and daughter tend to exclude father from the conversation and he makes no attempt to join in, it may well be that this is what also happens at home. It is reasonable for the therapist to check this out. If so the question may be posed as to whether everyone is happy with this and if not what alternatives may be sought.

The therapist may also ask the family to carry out an activity or task to illustrate some aspect of the way the family is structured and works. This might involve problem solving or decision making and again can provide useful information about how the family functions. Furthermore it is a step toward resolving difficulties.

When the therapist is uncertain about what is happening or how to proceed it is quite in order to share that uncertainty or simply to describe what appears to be happening. Similarly, it is unacceptable for therapists either to describe their own reactions to what is happening or to check, without sharing those reactions, whether family members have similar feelings.

It is helpful to focus on family roles and tasks, giving particular consideration to the cohesiveness and consistency of the parenting (see "Parental counselling" above). Not infrequently there is breaching of cross-generational boundaries so that a child and parent have an overclose relationship at the expense of the other parent and child(ren). The therapist would draw attention to this, explore its acceptability, try to understand what purpose it serves, and help the family decide how to proceed. It is quite reasonable to ask parents to sit next to each other in the sessions, if only because this makes it easier for the therapist to talk to them both at the same time. However it also highlights the importance of their working together as a parental team.

When parents complain that they have no control over a small child, for example when a father feels unable to prevent his 3 year old son from getting into danger, a useful technique is to ask the parent to stand next to the child. Their respective sizes are compared and the question asked why it is that the child cannot be protected.

Another helpful technique, which has some similarities to the family tree, is to ask family members to draw a family circle. This involves each person portraying within a circle their perceptions of the family, by including representations (for example their name) of each family member. The diagrams may illustrate closeness and distance, alliances and coalitions and power relationships within the family. The diagrams often highlight important discrepancies in perceptions, which can then be constructively explored.

Communication patterns

The way in which family members communicate with each other may be a significant contributor to difficulties. There are a number of communication dysfunctions:

- Little is said and there are prolonged periods of silence; problems are neither discussed nor resolved.
- One person does most of the talking, or acts as a "switchboard operator" channelling all communications, or appears to know what others are thinking (mind-reader).
- There is excessive communication, so that it appears as if everyone is talking at the same time and no one listens to anyone else. Alternatively one or more people talk at great length so that no one else can speak or the thread of what is being said is lost.

- There is a lack of congruence between verbal and non-verbal communication. A sad piece of information is more usually conveyed with sad affect. But non-congruence (i.e. the sad information is conveyed with a smile, or someone says "I am not angry" but looks and sounds angry) leads to confusion and eventually demoralisation.
- Thoughts and feelings are expressed by behaviour and physical symptoms rather than with words. A child who is fearful of school may have headaches on school mornings and the parents may therefore respond to the headache rather than the fears.

The therapy can focus quite specifically on the dysfunctional communication patterns. For example, in a family where communication is excessive, the therapist might suggest that each person takes a turn to say what he or she needs to, without interruption by others but nor at excessive length. The therapist then encourages brief responses to the specific points made, again without interruption. Gradually the family learn a more constructive communication style, which allows decisions to be made and problems to be solved. Different techniques are available for different styles, but the basic principles of ensuring each person is heard and acknowledged are the same.

Much the same can be said for the way in which families process feelings. These may spill out in a haphazard and chaotic way, or may be completely contained, or discouraged. The therapist assesses the family style and then encourages a direct sharing of feelings. There doesn't have to be agreement, but there does have to be an acknowledgement that the feelings exist and an acceptance that each person is entitled to their feelings, however unreasonable they may seem. Once people have a sense of being heard and accepted they can begin to think about change. The therapist's task is to support this process.

Indications for family therapy

Originally family therapy was mainly used in adult psychiatry. However, it is now most commonly used when children are presented by parents for help with mental health problems and indications include:

- Advice, reassurance and more basic counselling have failed to address the problem.
- The nature of the problem is less significant than the way the family is handling the problem.
- Where parents and children are having difficulty working together on the problems that face them.
- Where the nature of the problem requires a fundamental readjustment which the family have been unable to make to date.
- Medical disorders in which psychological factors play an important role, especially recurrent or chronic illness including asthma, diabetes, cystic fibrosis, and epilepsy. It is of particular relevance where treatment adherence has been problematic or response to treatment has been less than might reasonably be expected.
- Behavioural and emotional problems in the child requiring a clear, combined parental strategy. School refusal, separation anxiety, phobias, soiling and disruptive disorders fall into this category.
- The spectrum of child abuse and neglect.

Contraindications to family therapy

Lack of consent

Except in very unusual legal situations families should not be coerced into therapy.

Where there are threats to safety

If therapy threatens the safety of the therapist or any member of the family it should not proceed. Therapy is no substitute for protection.

Potential difficulties for family therapists

There are a number of problems that may complicate family therapy (Box 22.1). Most of these difficulties can either be

Box 22.1 Problems that may complicate family treatment

1 The parents use the treatment as a coercive opportunity to control the child. The clinician becomes an agent of the family and threatens the young person's autonomy or privacy

2 The clinician forms a strong alliance with one part of the family against the other and worsens the situation for the referred patient

3 The clinician fails to gain the trust and credibility of the family. The family may continue with reluctance or even discontinue

4 The family wants to be given support, instead of making changes. They become dependent upon the clinician

5 The family wants resolution of the presenting problem when change is not possible and acceptance is necessary. They become angry because the clinician has not "fixed" the problem

6 The family sees no connection between what is happening in the family as a whole and what the child is experiencing. They remain fixed on "the symptom"

7 A key family member (usually the father) fails to attend and therefore blocks the possibility of problem resolution

8 Blaming parents for all that has happened but failing to mobilise them to take control or contribute to the direction of the family in the future. Parents feel guilty and are unable to acknowledge errors or work on change

9 The therapist has an individual relationship with everyone in the family, but fails to relate to them as a family unit and to address what is happening between members

10 The therapist is put in the role which the child previously fulfilled and is blamed for the family's problems

11 The treatment goes on without clear goals or purpose

avoided or overcome by careful reflection about the therapy. Supervision is particularly important for the less experienced therapists but even the more experienced can benefit. Sticking to basics rather than trying to be too clever helps to minimise many problems. Box 22.2 lists some points to be considered for avoiding some of the pitfalls.

Therapy tends to end gradually and often before there is complete resolution of difficulties. This is not unreasonable, as long as the family are on the right course. The parents' needs and wishes will generally take precedence and as long as the children's well being is assured this should be respected. By contrast, if there has been no change over a period of several months and there seems little prospect of change then a different therapy or a different therapist may be indicated.

Box 22.2 Pitfalls in family therapy

1 Be wary of trying to be a better "parent" in the therapy than the parents. Be an example but not a competitor
2 Avoid blaming the parents. Parents do make mistakes but it pays to be humble and to acknowledge a common tendency to error
3 Be careful not to see everything from one person's point of view, either parent or child
4 Don't see every problem as due to the family system. Poverty, disease and bad luck also play their part. Not all causality is circular or interactional. If a child is intellectually impaired, the direction of causality is not bidirectional in the same sense as it is for many other problems. Implications that the child is impaired by the family interactions are cruel and incorrect
5 Distinguish between the biological system of the family's bodies and the meaning system of their minds. They are to some extent linked but also separate systems
6 Pay attention to safety issues such as violence, abuse, suicidal threats, and failure to adhere to medication
7 Don't socialise with family members
8 Respect the privacy of each family member
9 Avoid getting caught up in a marital conflict
10 Don't take responsibility for removing a problem from a family
11 There is no need to be defensive about not having children, being single, or being younger than some family members. Experience is helpful but not essential and the therapist's prime task is to help the family find their own solutions rather than providing them for the family
12 Distinguish between difficulties that belong to the family in treatment as opposed to oneself

Conclusion

Helping parents and families is not a mystical set of arcane skills limited to those who have been trained by gurus. It is a practical approach to being helpful to those who are of importance to the child or young person in distress and an essential part of psychiatric treatment for this age group. Treatment ranges from basic support and advice through to quite intensive family therapy. Such an approach is ultimately a very complex set of skills based on the notion that the only way to understand a part of anything is to consider the whole.

Further reading

Carr A. *Family therapy*. Chichester: John Wiley, 2000.

Hoffman L. *Family therapy*. New York: WW Norton, 2001.

Lask J, Maynard C. Engaging and working with the family. In: Green J, Jacobs B, eds. *In-patient child psychiatry—Modern practice, research and the future*. London: Routledge, 1998:75–92.

23: Psychotherapy

Introduction

There are many different types of psychotherapy based upon many different beliefs and premises, but they have many characteristics in common. The biggest cluster of psychotherapy types, prior to the cognitive therapy revolution, might be loosely described as psychodynamic. This chapter introduces the general principles of individual child psychotherapy with a special emphasis on psychodynamic psychotherapy, while chapter 24 will deal with cognitive behavioural psychotherapy. (It is worth emphasising here that there can be considerable overlap between the psychotherapies. The distinction is to some extent artificial, especially nowadays when clinicians and therapists draw upon a number of different theoretical models for their clinical practice.) The aim of this chapter is to enable clinicians to apply the broad principles of psychotherapy to any clinical encounter and also to enable more informed referral behaviour to colleagues who are specialist psychotherapists.

The cluster of psychodynamic psychotherapies have a number of beliefs in common:

- *Talking with and listening to patients can be therapeutic.*
- *Talking and listening are most helpful when they occur in the context of a relationship—the therapeutic relationship.*
- *The relationships that are most therapeutic are open, honest, and based upon trust.*
- *These characteristics can be built into a professional helping situation.* This can only happen if:
  - The relationship is clearly distinguished from non-professional relationships—i.e. a professional boundary is established. The relationship is clearly defined in terms of when, where, and how frequently the patient will be seen, i.e. a boundary or limit is set to the demands of the relationship.
  - The focus is on the needs of the patient not those of the therapist.

Some clinicians also stipulate a fixed number of sessions at the end of which the therapy will cease. These agreed arrangements are often referred to as the treatment alliance— the therapeutic contract or understanding that exists between clinician and patient. When therapy is offered for a child or young adolescent it will be wholly or partly negotiated with the parents, depending upon the developmental maturity of the young person.

- *There are forces (hence the word dynamic) for change and for resisting change within the patient, of which the patient is unaware.* Those negative forces inhibiting change are sometimes labelled "resistance".
- *What happens in one part of the patient's life or one time in the patient's life is connected with the rest of the patient's life.* When there are repeated themes over time in relationships it is sometimes referred to as the compulsion to repeat or "the repetition compulsion". When there is a connection between one part of patients' lives and their relationship with the clinician it is called transference. Transference is particularly used when patients have a distorted perspective of the relationship based on another part of their lives. When there is the same sort of connection between a part of the clinician's life and the treatment relationship it is referred to as counter-transference. These phenomena are based upon the tendency to generalise from one part of our experience to another and that this is done largely subconsciously. Sometimes in the process of generalising from previous experience, the actual situation is obscured by these other experiences. For example, a previously abused child may become terrified by a therapist who asks about why a treatment session was missed, or a therapist may feel saddened or angered when a teenager reveals struggles of a similar kind to those experienced by the therapist earlier in life.
- *Making sense of what is happening in our feelings, behaviour and relationships is likely to give us a greater sense of control and a reduction in our internal conflicts.* Some therapists believe it is the making sense of experience that makes the difference. Others feel it is the nature of the relationship between the clinician and the patient that makes the

difference. However all are agreed that making sense and the treatment relationship are critical ingredients. Persisting with treatment through all the difficulties faced within and outside the treatment setting is called "working through". It sometimes involves dealing with hundreds of examples of situations before the patient sees their tendency to unwittingly distort reality. Gradually the patient learns to see situations as they are and not as they fear or wish them to be.

- *Good treatment may include the patient being disappointed with the clinician but still maintaining a basic trust and persisting with the therapy.* Clinicians are not perfect. The patient's ability to accept the limitations and imperfections can be a helpful experience. Accepting our own limitations and imperfections is referred to by some therapists as "the depressive position". It does not mean becoming clinically depressed. It means maturing psychologically to the point where we realise that the world of our experience and ourselves are not simply good or bad, black or white, right or wrong. We relinquish fairytale worlds to accept our more ambiguous, less clear cut and morally grey universe.

- *That some people find therapy that aims at understanding too troubling, too confronting, and too overwhelming.* Those who have had too many troubles, too little nurture, too few supports and too much pain are likely to require support, succour, encouragement and helpful advice about how to get through the next set of problems that face them. Understanding the "why" of their problems is like holding up a mirror to a trauma victim. It may only increase the distress. Supportive psychotherapy focuses on isolating the present experience to the "here and now", not generalising back to the "there and then". The aim is relief and support not probing and understanding. Therapists make a distinction between "insight oriented psychotherapy" and "supportive psychotherapy". If we give insight oriented therapy to the wrong people they may become anxious, overwhelmed and their emotional state and behaviour may deteriorate. If we give supportive therapy to the wrong people they may become overly reliant on us to help them. Children and young people almost always require a combination of both, given that they are prone to become overwhelmed and overly reliant.

- *Certain themes occur frequently in psychotherapy:*
  - trust and mistrust
  - control and loss of control
  - closeness and distance
  - dependence and independence
  - openness and privacy
  - anger and love
  - insecurity and safety
  - anxiety and hope
  - sexuality and boundaries
  - expectation and disappointment
  - loss and despair.

- *The ability to cope with loss is an essential part of living and loving.* The ending of therapy is a critical part of the therapy. Most therapists have the end of therapy clearly in mind from the day they say hello. Mini-separations like therapist holidays, missed treatment sessions or times of illness provide opportunities to prepare for these issues.

Who might benefit?

There are prerequisites for this sort of therapy. A normal IQ is helpful but not essential. However, those who are in the moderate intellectual disability range and below are not usually able to make use of this sort of therapy. Children with marked receptive speech difficulties will require more play and less talk. When receptive speech difficulties are combined with social and emotional impairment the child is less likely to benefit. A child who has an unstable home placement and who has no permanency plan is prone to confuse therapy with placement. So too are some of those who refer. The presence of distress is not the justification for psychotherapy. This is akin to confusing the presence of pain with the need for an operation. An operation may cause pain and complicate. So, too, inappropriate psychotherapy may generate more distress, confuse and complicate an already difficult situation, not to mention diverting much needed resources to no good end. Those who benefit most from psychodynamic psychotherapy are those whose:

- Verbal skills are adequate
- Emotional state is stable but distressing
- Parents' and home situation are supportive, even if the family are uncertain as to how they might help.

What sort of psychotherapy? (Table 23.1)

In practice most young people need a combination of support, understanding and teaching, but more troubled and traumatised children need more support and teaching and less focus on understanding emotions and relationships. Chapter 24 is about therapy that teaches how to think differently—cognitive behavioural therapy.

How to be supportive

Take time to listen, validate and empathise with the child's distress but then focus on how they managed, what they are doing right, and what strengths they have. It is a fine line sometimes between focusing on strengths and failing to empathise with distress. Humour can be very helpful but is always in danger of being interpreted as "not taking me seriously" if carried too far.

It is important to keep short term expectations low in very troubled teenagers but long term expectations moderate and specific:

> We may not be able to remove all your "pain", but we will be able to help you live with your pain a little better ... We will not be able to take away all of the emptiness or boredom you feel, but we will help you to handle the emptiness inside you better ... We will not be able to eliminate the "waves of distress" that often make you act impulsively or on the spur of the moment when you do things to get relief or feel tormented and agitated, but this treatment will help you to see that "this too will pass" and you can survive it without resorting to inappropriate behaviours.

Finally, we aim for brief interviews only (half an hour is usually enough), not too frequently (fortnightly or monthly is sufficient for longer term patients), and we emphasise termination but approach this gradually when dependency is intense.

Table 23.1 What are the differences between providing support, providing understanding of emotions, and teaching how to change thinking

Psychotherapy which aims to support	Psychotherapy which aims to explain emotions and relationships	Psychotherapy which teaches how to change thinking
For those with fewer psychological strengths and more broad ranging vulnerability	For those with more strengths, more backup, more resilience and who want to make sense of their relationships and feelings	For those who prefer to approach things through a thinking, educational and skills based approach
Concentrates on coping, strengths and solving particular problems. Getting through difficult times with the skills they have rather than learning new skills	Concentrates on areas of struggle, vulnerability, sensitivity, and relationships. Patterns of relating are identified across different relationships and different stages of life	Concentrates on unrealistic thinking patterns about themselves, their world, and their future. Problem solving goes beyond the particular problem to the way similar problems are solved using a particular problem as a model
Focuses on what is happening "here and now" in the room and their lives	Focuses on what happened "there and then" in their past linked to "out there in their relationships"	Focuses on what is happening "here and now" in their heads and their lives but does so with special reference to particular thoughts and feelings and how these might be challenged

(Continued)

Table 23.1 (*Continued*)

Psychotherapy which aims to support	Psychotherapy which aims to explain emotions and relationships	Psychotherapy which teaches how to change thinking
Aim of therapy is supporting the child or young person to keep going, as they are, as well as possible, by encouragement, advice, and regular sessions	Aim of therapy is to change the child or young person's style of coping, feeling and relating by changing their view of all their relationships by the therapeutic relationship	Aim of therapy is to change the child or young person's style of coping, feeling and relating by teaching them a more practical thinking style
Main therapeutic skill is to foster confidence in their own coping capacity	Main therapeutic skill is to give understanding as to why they feel as they do	Main therapeutic skill is to show them how the way they think affects the way they feel and teaching them how to think more helpfully

Emergencies should be dealt with pragmatically, sympathetically, and supportively. For example, the focus of work with a chronically suicidal adolescent should be on enhancing coping skills.

How to be understanding

There are four main skills that promote understanding:

- Exploring vulnerability sensitively
- Linking experiences thoughtfully
- Using images and metaphors creatively
- Reiterating themes persistently.

Exploring vulnerability sensitively

Warmth, empathy, non-judgmental acceptance, and genuine non-burdensome self-disclosure, humour and hope have all been shown to be non-specifically therapeutic. These are prerequisites of all good therapists whether they are cognitive, behavioural, family or pharmacotherapists. Nevertheless they are especially needed in the task of exploring the vulnerable inner world of the child or adolescent.

A helpful technique is to explore the anxieties the young person has in relation to the interview before dealing with sensitive or painful feelings. For example if a young "person" is reluctant to speak avoiding eye contact:

Clinician: It's sometimes hard to talk about things that are very personal [focusing on difficulties relating in the interview].

The young person looks sad and tearful and acknowledges it by a nod.

Clinician: You seem very upset … You look quite sad … [exploring and clarifying the feelings].

The young person begins to talk a little and it becomes clear that she is angry at being let down by friends and rejected by a boyfriend.

Clinician: Sometimes, I get sad when I'm hurt by others ... when I'm really angry that other people have let me down [identifying the longer term issues of anger and reliance on friends].

This shift from style of relating in the interview, to current emotional state then to addressing longer term issues of attitude, need and turmoil enables sensitive issues to be addressed gently and almost seamlessly.

Linking experience thoughtfully

There are many types of linkages:

- *Past and present experiences.* What is happening here and now seems to be linked to what has happened previously?
- *Present relationships with other relationships.* What is happening at home and what is happening at school?
- *Therapeutic relationships with other relationships.* What is happening "inside therapy" is linked to what is happening "outside therapy"?
- *One part of therapy with another.* A child might draw a particular theme that links to something discussed earlier.
- *Behaviour and predicament.* Sometimes a child may graphically represent in their behaviour or bodily symptoms a psychological theme in their lives, for example non-organic blindness in someone locked in denial.
- *Combinations of the above.* Sometimes many linkages occur simultaneously; there may be similarities between what is happening in the therapy, at home, at school, and in the past.

Suggestions for linkages   Linkages should not be made lightly or coercively. Some therapists make linkages in an artificial way, and others too often or too quickly. As a general rule:

- Attempt partial and simple linkages before full, combined or complicated linkages.
- Get the facts straight and know the patient before jumping to premature linkages.

- Give room for the child or adolescent to disagree or refuse the linkage.
- Beware of the overly compliant child who agrees with any interpretation or linkage.
- Therapists should be wary of their own favourite interpretations. These may be more to do with the therapist's own issues than those of the child.
- Getting an interpretation wrong can make a child feel misunderstood. Be ready to acknowledge errors rather than interpreting their unwillingness to accept it as resistance.
- Track the responses to linkages—not just the immediate response but also later. Links that are powerful are not static. Growing anger and resentment may follow initial acceptance. Initial resentment and denial may be followed by growing relief and appreciation.
- Don't confuse what is happening in the real world with what is happening in the young person. An example of an unhelpful comment would be: "Perhaps you made yourself get sick with asthma". On the other hand: "Sometimes when we become ill there can be good spin offs ... can you see any good things coming out of you being ill?" could be helpful.

Using images and metaphor creatively

Any communication is based on using symbols and gestures for parts of our experience. Words are just such symbols. Clinicians are thinking all the time of how to capture key aspects of a child's experience in vivid picture symbols, words, and gestures. Play, drawings, sculpting, stories and drama may all capture important themes. Perhaps what is most important to the child is that an adult is trying to help; trying to understand; trying to alleviate distress.

Reiterating themes

Most of us learn by rehearsal, reiteration, exposure, and re-exposure. Patterns of behaving, feeling and relating are not easily changed, but children and adolescents are more accessible than adults to change. The same message may need to be retold in countless different situations and in numerous ways before it leads to positive change. Good clinicians persist creatively and hopefully rather than polemically and resignedly.

What can a child and their parents expect from psychotherapy?

Where will I have therapy?

Fortunately children are flexible and almost any room will do as long as privacy is assured. Generally the therapist will use the same rooms to give them a sense of stability and predictability. Most therapists have a room with interesting and fun play materials.

How often will I be seen?

Most therapists see children once a week initially and then make a decision whether or not to increase. It is often better to meet less frequently and to increase than vice versa. Most families find more than twice a week difficult to sustain. Most children find less than once a fortnight too infrequent to sustain continuity. "Tough times" may warrant some extra sessions, but this is usually done thoughtfully.

How long is each session?

The standard answer with adults is 50 minutes. However, some children will only be able to tolerate 15–20 minutes, while others can cope with longer. Some may need a break in the session and therapists should take into account the child's ability to concentrate, tolerate intimacy, and emotional intensity.

How many sessions?

Most therapists need to three to six sessions to assess suitability for psychotherapy. Most give one or two sessions weekly for at least 3 months and rarely more than 2 years. Three months is the minimum period for human adaptation to a major developmental trauma while 2 years is the period after which most experiential responses are regarded as chronic or long term. This means that with sessions once a week, therapy will rarely be fewer than 12 sessions with most therapies being about 20–40 sessions. This may have as much to do with therapist availability as it is with child need.

What is the basic structure of the therapy?

Assessment
3–6 sessions: assessment for suitability

Engagement
4–10 sessions: settling in and building trust

Working through
10–20 sessions: getting into the big issues and coming to grips with basic styles of behaving, feeling, and relating

Finishing up
4–10 sessions: reexperiencing the early symptoms of fears of their return. Facing issues of separation and loss

What is the basic structure of an individual session?

Warming up
What has happened since we last met?

Loosening up
What will we talk about and do today?

Facing up
Facing something new about myself, the past, and the future

Finishing up
Getting ready to leave the therapist and to go back to daily life

When will therapy end?

- When the child's distress has been reduced.
- When the child has developed effective coping skills.

The therapist will discuss finishing long before it happens. It will not be sprung on the child and family without notice.

Some key points about psychotherapy

The characteristics of the good child psychotherapist, the problems that may complicate individual psychotherapy and a list of "don'ts" when talking with children are given in Boxes 23.1–23.3 respectively.

Box 23.1 Characteristics of the good child psychotherapist

1. Trained in working with children
2. A genuine care for children
3. Know who they can and cannot help and the limits of the therapy
4. Willing to liaise closely with colleagues
5. Able to communicate with parents in a way that does not make them feel locked out while still ensuring the confidentiality of the child
6. Willing to open their work to colleague scrutiny and support
7. The ability to apply the general principles to day to day, informal therapeutic interactions
8. The ability to see children's strengths as well as their vulnerability
9. An awareness of the subtleties of the way things happening in the real world may interact with what happens in the child's inner world
10. Open to having got it wrong and to new information
11. A concern for the entire well being of the child including ensuring medical factors are considered in their care
12. Able to see that other factors may contribute to the child's well being
13. Willing to collaborate with other therapies such as family therapy, medication, and educational interventions
14. Sees the child's need to do without them

Everyone has problems and concerns. Therapy aims to help children and young people deal with their problems differently and less stressfully, rather than turn them into 'perfect' human beings.

What should the parents be told

Parents need to know their child is safe and being managed professionally. They have a right to know things that they

Box 23.2 Problems that may complicate individual psychotherapy

1. A parent may give partial or fluctuating consent
2. Parents may fail to support the child's therapy in terms of time, transport, or attitude to therapy
3. A parent may be envious of or competitive with the child for the therapy
4. The therapist may unthinkingly or unwittingly support the role of the parent
5. The therapist may allow a therapy to proceed where placement has not been clarified
6. The therapist may become overidentified with the child against the parents
7. The therapist may become an agent of parental control over the child
8. Therapy may be terminated prematurely or without sufficient preparation
9. Therapy may be prolonged unnecessarily
10. The child may deteriorate in the course of therapy and fail to reintegrate as therapy proceeds
11. Therapists may find themselves unable to like and engage with the child or vice versa
12. Therapists may find they are unable to say goodbye

Box 23.3 Don'ts when talking with children

1. Don't confuse your role with that of a parent
2. Don't use your developmental, linguistic or intellectual superiority to coerce the child
3. Don't confuse your role with that of a playmate
4. Don't try to be too clever
5. Don't use long, complicated, jargon-laden and ideologically based sentences
6. Don't rush the interview
7. Don't strain the child's concentration
8. Don't keep asking questions
9. Don't be afraid of helpful discipline that ensures safety
10. Don't burden the child with your problems
11. Don't compete with parents for the child's affection and understanding
12. Don't be afraid to acknowledge what you don't understand

could do to help their child move on in resolving their difficulties. They have a right to have a broad understanding of the purpose and progress of therapy, but not the detailed content. It is also important to explain the need for the child to be assured of confidentiality unless there is a threat to the safety of the child. Safety always trumps confidentiality.

Conclusion

Psychotherapy, whilst not simple, is based on simple rational principles. Many of these should be applied throughout clinical practice, others should be reserved for a more formal psychotherapeutic relationship. Psychotherapy varies in its aims and style, from the offering of support through to in depth exploration of subconscious material. The skilled clinician will be familiar with the basic principles and use them naturally but will also be aware of when and why to refer.

Further reading

Axline V. *Dibs: in search of self.* Ringwood, Australia: Penguin, 1979.
Carr A. *Handbook of child and adolescent psychology—a contextual approach.* London: Routledge, 1999.
Freud A. *Introduction to the technique of child analysis* (1926–27). Reprinted in: *The psychoanalytic treatment of children.* London: Imago Press, 1946 [advanced reading].
Malan D. *Individual psychotherapy and the new science of psychodynamics.* Sydney: Butterworths, 1998 [advanced reading].

24: Cognitive behavioural therapy

Introduction

Helping children with their thoughts and behaviour has become highly technical with specific treatments for specific disorders. However many of the treatments are based on principles articulated by ancient philosophers and theologians. Many wise clinicians do practice cognitive behavioural therapy (CBT) without realising it. CBT was developed largely in adult practice and although there are problems in transposing that experience to children and adolescents, much has been gained in so doing. Key ideas in CBT are outlined in Box 24.1 (see also Table 23.1).

Box 24.1 Key ideas in cognitive behavioural therapy

- The human condition is not explained by describing behaviour and feelings alone. Understanding thinking throws essential light on behaviour and feelings
- Thinking affects feelings and behaviour
- Changing thinking changes feelings and behaviour
- Different thoughts and styles of thinking affect vulnerability to distressing feelings and undesirable behaviours

---

The way we think when bad and good things happen

1A: When bad things happen, a tendency to believe that they will keep happening, or that their impact will be permanent and unchangeable, increases depressive feelings and behaviours. This might be called the Humpty Dumpty thought—the belief that all the King's horses and all the King's men cannot put Humpty together again.

1B: When good things happen, a tendency to believe that they will be short lived and subject to change, reduces positive feelings and behaviours. This is the belief that good things are merely "5 minutes of sunshine".

2A: When bad things happen in one area of our lives a tendency to believe that they will happen, or have an impact, on most areas of our lives, increases depressive feelings and behaviours. Like a pack of cards, when one falls there is a cascade.

2B: When good things happen in one area of our lives, a tendency to believe that good things and their impact, will be confined or restricted to that part of our lives, reduces positive feelings or behaviours. Good things may be confined to one part of the mind with little impact on the rest of our experience.

3A: When bad things happen, a tendency to believe they happen to me in particular, and that somehow I contributed to it, increases depressive feelings and behaviours. This personalising of all adversity has a particularly corrosive effect on self-esteem.

3B: When good things happen, a tendency to believe they happen to everybody, and that it was merely luck or someone else's good judgement, rather than any contribution on our part, reduces positive feelings or behaviours. This disownership of success and good fortune makes a turn of events for the better lacking in benefit.

4: When bad things happen and we attempt to avoid them, we can come to rely on avoidance as our main strategy for solving problems. Anxiety is the effect we experience when we believe that avoidance is the only way to stop current bad things happening.

Therapeutic principles

- If children can learn a set of unhelpful beliefs they can unlearn them.
- Therapy involves transforming:
  - passive suffering into active problem solving

- implicit assumptions into explicit issues that can be debated between therapist and young person
- a non-articulated apprehension into a verbalised and identified threat that can then be addressed.

- Therapy involves fragmenting our negative generalisations about ourselves, our world and our futures and unifying our positive generalisations.
- Removal of negatively distorted beliefs makes living more manageable and coping is improved.

Who is suitable for CBT?

If the child has had difficulties in thinking for any reason, therapies that rely on the ability to think clearly are unlikely to be helpful. Those children who find this therapy helpful are usually verbal or, if hearing impaired, capable of signing. They usually require a normal intellectual level. They also require the ability to make generalisations about the sort of person they are, the sort of world they live in, and the sort of future they have. This is unusual before the age of 7 years and in most intellectually normal children is present by the age of 10 years.

In addition, some children and adolescents prefer the less emotionally focused and more educational approach of CBT, to the non-directive, affectively probing approach of psychodynamic psychotherapy.

It is always worth remembering the "B" in CBT. Behavioural therapies are able to be used in the non-verbal, the intellectually impaired, and even the neonate. This chapter concentrates on the cognitive components but throughout the book extensive reference is made to behavioural principles and techniques.

Characteristics of the good cognitive behavioural therapist

The 12 characteristics that the good cognitive behaviour therapist should possess are listed in Box 24.2.

Box 24.2 Twelve characteristics of the good cognitive behavioural therapist

1. Be an active listener
2. Respect other clinicians involved in the care and management of a child
3. Make the concepts of CBT simple, clear and practical for the child
4. Accurately feed back to the child their own thoughts, feelings and behaviours so that they might feel understood
5. Creatively develop exercises, homework and graduated approaches to feared situations that match and extend the child's coping style
6. Reassure parents that the time the child spends with the therapist does not undermine the parents' place and role in the child's life
7. Teach parents to be "therapists" on behalf of the child and to utilise the therapeutic principles in their parenting
8. Integrate "non-specific" therapeutic characteristics (such as warmth, hope, acceptance, compassion, humour) with specific CBT skills
9. Educate without dominating. This is particularly important where children have had negative educational experiences
10. Identify the elements of readiness for therapy in both the child and the parents (distress with the symptoms, concern about educational and personal impact in the short and long term, and understanding of the connection between the treatments and the disorder)
11. Reduce the number of issues being dealt with at any one time to one or two at most
12. Know when to say "goodbye" and when to have "booster" sessions to remotivate, re-educate and reorientate towards change

Contraindications to CBT

- The non-verbal child who is unable to sign.
- Intellectual disability (mild disability in older teenagers is a grey zone).
- Children below 7 years of age.
- Parental unwillingness for the child to be seen individually. This is an indicator to offer CBT in the family context.
- Anything that impairs thinking such as medical illness, physical exhaustion, severe depression, delirium, psychosis, and dementia. CBT for psychosis is being developed but requires particular skills.

Practical CBT techniques

Teaching children and adolescents:

- How to tell the difference between thoughts, feelings, and bodily symptoms:
  - Thought spotting—may be hard in younger children.
  - Feeling finding—giving the feeling words. Exercises such as watching movies where emotions are exemplified and role playing may be helpful.
  - Symptom searches—talking about which parts of the body feel what is helpful and often illuminating in children who somatise.

Each of these skills requires the creative use of drawings, rating scales, videos, family photograph albums, and other visual and tactile media.

- To be detectives or scientists, searching for evidence with their own thoughts.
- To be judge and jury in weighing up the evidence of their own thinking.
- To disagree with their own thinking when they can see that it is not based on evidence.
- To face fears—avoidance can be a self-defeating strategy and fears can be overcome gradually. This means taking a situation that is only feared slightly and finding an approach to overcoming it. Moving through a hierarchy of feared situations from least to most, gives increasing confidence for facing the worst fears and tackling the most entrenched avoidance.
- To see that solution-finding skills gradually need to replace problem-generating skills.
- To accept what can and cannot be changed and reducing the expenditure of wasted energy on the insoluble.
- To try to remain relaxed and lower "the emotional temperature", to enable clear thinking and constructive listening and talking.
- To discuss fears without being frightened and to gain mastery over them.
- Social skills—what to do and say in various situations. This is combined with dealing with unhelpful thoughts about

what others may be thinking: "He is quiet because he thinks I'm dumb".

- Appropriate assertiveness—not to think of themselves as inferior, "doormats", or always having to yield to others' assessments of them.
- To praise themselves when they have done the right thing.
- To allow for imperfection and occasional failures.

These strategies help to restructure the young person's thinking. Behind them is the underpinning assumption that coping can be taught and hoping can be justified. CBT is deeply optimistic, thoroughly educational in approach, and always practical.

Here are also some areas of "don'ts" in CBT:

- Neglect the parents.
- Rush into providing CBT before helping the parents to feel comfortable with it.
- Encourage the parent to expect that CBT will address *all* problems the child faces.
- "Preach" CBT to the parents and child. It is a treatment method rather than an ideology.
- Be impatient in finding a solution: detective work takes time and involves listening.
- Denigrate other therapies that might be helpful in addition to CBT.
- Forget that CBT will have failures, as do all forms of therapies.
- Blame the patient if the treatment does not work.
- Assume that the treatment will never work if it does not work at first. Other treatments, time and improvement in the illness may make the child or family more prepared for CBT.
- Give up when standard approaches fail. Think of more creative ways to address the same issue.
- Confuse cognitive changes with emotional and behavioural changes. Cognition is the means, but emotional and behavioural change are still the goals.
- Try to do too many things in the one session.
- Become too complicated—keep it simple.

A brief word about the "B" in CBT

The more recent enthusiasm for cognitive approaches should not cause us to forget older behavioural therapies and their possible benefits when used with children.

Indications

Behavioural therapy is particularly of value when a child's thoughts are difficult to assess. The non-verbal or inarticulate child with learning difficulties deserves special consideration for this sort of therapy. However, it is also of value in otherwise normal children, especially in the under sevens, where cognitive approaches may still demand too much developmentally. The more discrete and context specific the undesirable behaviour is the more likely the behaviour will respond to rewards. The more diffuse the symptom and the more generalised to different contexts, the less likely is there to be a clear favourable outcome.

The principal method of treatment

However technical or complex, the main method of being helpful is to reward desirable behaviour and not to reward undesirable behaviour. Proximity in time to the desirable behaviour is important.

The principal explanation of undesirable behaviour

The purpose of analysing the child's behaviour is to identify the reward—seeking the nature or function of the behaviour. This will usually fall into five reward categories—stimulus, company, care, approval, and things valued by the child. They correspond to behaviours to avoid boredom, loneliness, neglect, rejection, and dispossession.

The principal difficulties

All forms of treatment require application of the principles and some consistency. Parental behaviour is one of the most powerful rewards and sometimes parents may, unwittingly, find powerful rewards in some of their children's behaviours. This provides the classic basis for a vicious behavioural cycle. A child's distress may elicit care which in turn may relieve the child's distress. The child may then become more distressed to obtain more relief. Parents are naturally reluctant to refuse to relieve their child's distress. They are often only willing to consider on the basis that we have to be "cruel to be kind".

The place of behavioural therapy

Behavioural principles underlie all other therapies. If any form of interviewing is habitually aversive, avoidant behaviour will result. If praise and reward are not used to good effect most therapies will fail. In the intellectually impaired and the very young child, behavioural therapies and parental advice on behavioural principles are the mainstay of treatment. Predictability of, and approval by, therapists remain powerful reinforcers in any therapy.

Conclusion

CBT offers a simple, practical and solution-focused approach to many problems. It is of most value for those children with problems such as depression, anxiety disorders and obsessive compulsive disorder. Attention deficit hyperactivity disorder and problems with anger control have responded well to CBT. It should always be accompanied by a thoughtful understanding of the behavioural factors contributing to the symptoms from both the child and the parents. Almost all clinicians now include some cognitive and behavioural principles in their work. Good clinicians probably always have.

Further reading

Rapee RM, Spence SH, Cobham V, Wignall A. *Helping your anxious child: a step by step guide for parents*, Sydney: New Harbinger Publications, 2000.

Rapee RM, Wignall A, Hidsen JL, Schniering CA. *Anxious children and adolescents: an evidence-based approach.* Sydney: New Harbinger Publications, 2000.

Seligman MEP,Reivich K, Jaycox L, Gilham J. *The optimistic child.* Sydney: Random House Press, 1985.

Tanner S, Ball J. *Beating the blues: a self-help approach to overcoming depression.* Sydney: Doubleday, 1989.

25: Psychopharmacology

Introduction

The revolution of pharmacological discovery that changed the face of adult psychiatry occurred in the decade 1949–60 with the discovery of many of the main types of psychotropic agents. It is only in the last decade that the broad variety of these agents has begun to be available for children suffering from mental illness. There is a growing body of evidence for efficacy in this age group. However, like so many treatments in the paediatric age range, much has to be initially extrapolated from adulthood while experience and evidence are gathered. This chapter is a distillation of information likely to be of benefit to the busy clinician aiming to add medication to comprehensive child psychiatric treatment or to consider possible adverse effects in its usage.

The general principles for the use of psychotropics in childhood are listed in Box 25.1.

Indications for medication

There are now many conditions in childhood that may benefit from medication (Table 25.1). Traditionally medications have been used when non-biological therapies have failed. In milder conditions where distress is not extreme, containment and safety are not at issue, this seems reasonable. However, as

---

Box 25.1 General principles for the use of psychotropics in childhood

1. Start the dose low and increase slowly
2. Attempt monotherapy to begin with wherever possible
3. If polytherapy is being considered, discuss with a colleague and document the discussion
4. If introducing further psychotropics, do so one at a time in order to assess the impact of addition

5. If withdrawing a psychotropic, do so one at a time to assess the impact of subtraction
6. If changing the doses of medication when there are multiple psychotropics, do so one at a time to assess the impact of the change
7. Side effects are minimised by making changes slowly
8. Try to give an adequate trial in time (about 3 months) in an adequate dose (the highest tolerable and safe dose) before relinquishing it as without benefit. Most psychotropic medication is never given an adequate trial
9. Do not allow chaotic families to lead to chaotic prescribing
10. Better to use a small number of drugs regularly than to try many different kinds infrequently
11. Treat each case as a single case study and be sure what symptoms and signs you are targetting
12. Warn of the common and serious side effects
13. Parents who pressurise you to prescribe may also be the parents who will take you to court if things go wrong
14. Wherever possible review, audit and share your practice with a peer group and then document the discussion
15. In general avoid agonists and antagonists of the same neurotransmitter group
16. Where agonists or antagonists of the same neurotransmitter group are being used they should generally be targetting a different locus within the neurone, for example levodopa and bromocryptine both target the dopaminergic system but one is a substrate and the other targets postsynaptic receptors
17. Do not use combined agonists lightly, for example amitriptyline and thioridazine are powerful anticholinergic agonists
18. Do not use stimulants in psychosis
19. If a child has a primary problem with tics do not use stimulants for their inattention. If a child has a primary problem with attention and only a secondary or relatively minor problem with tics, consideration for stimulants may be given if alpha agonists are unsuccessful
20. Do not use the reversible inhibitors of the mono-oxidase A (RIMAs) and the selective serotonin reuptake inhibitors (SSRIs) together
21. Do not use SSRIs and tricyclics together
22. If discretion is given to families or older patients about altering dosage be very clear what the limits to the discretion are
23. Dentists should be warned about the use of epinephrine (adrenaline) in those on tricyclics and the noradrenergic reuptake inhibitors
24. Do not prescribe moclobemide to a known user of methylenedioxymethamphetamine (MDMA or "ecstasy")
25. If antipsychotic medication is required in children or young people always use atypically as a first line unless acute containment is necessary and regular monitoring for movement disorders is essential

Table 25.1 Indications of particular medication groups by condition

Indications by conditions	SSRIs and 5HT$_{2A}$ antagonists	Tricyclics	SNRIS	Benzodiazepines	Atypical antipsychotics	Typical antipsychotics	Lithium	Anticonvulsants	Stimulants	Alpha-2 agonists
Anxiety disorders	1st line: Sertraline Fluoxetine Paroxetine Citalopram Fluvoxamine Nefazadone	Amitriptyline	2nd line: Venlafaxine	Diazepam Alprazolam (short term only)	Occasionally in intellectually impaired may use risperidone or olanzapine to avoid disinhibition of benzodiazepines and akathisia of SSRIs	Occasionally in intellectually impaired may use thioridazine, usually short term	No	No	No	Clonidine mainly when anxiety accompanies post-traumatic stress disorders
Major depressive disorder ± melancholia	1st line: Sertraline Fluoxetine Paroxetine Fluvoxamine Nefazadone	Not effective in childhood and adolescence	2nd line: Venlafaxine	Diazepam for insomnia and agitation	Olanzapine, risperidone for psychotic depression	Only after atypicals have been used in psychosis. Sometimes used short term to supplement or for IV use	No	No	No	No
OCD	1st line: Fluvoxamine Sertraline Fluoxetine Paroxetine	2nd line: Clomipramine (some experts would still argue that this is 1st line)	Venlafaxine for combined depression and OCD	Clonazepam if sleep and agitation prominent	Olanzapine for extreme OCD. OCD has been recorded to be worsened in some people by the use of risperidone	If atypicals make worse or fail to improve in extreme OCD	In extreme OCD to augment tricyclics or SSRIs	No	No	It is not uncommon in Asperger's children to have symptoms of OCD, ADHD and tics. Clonidine may be used here as a 1st line
Tourette's syndrome	As above where comorbid OCD	Clomipramine where resistant	Rarely if inattention, OCD and	Clonazepam	1st line: Risperidone Olanzapine unless	2nd line: haloperidol, pimo-zide if OCD not	No	No	No	1st line for mild Tourette's with ADHD

(Continued)

Table 25.1 (Continued)

Indications by conditions	SSRIs and 5HT$_{2A}$ antagonists	Tricyclics	SNRIS	Benzodiazepines	Atypical antipsychotics	Typical antipsychotics	Lithium	Anticonvulsants	Stimulants	Alpha-2 agonists
		OCD also present	depression prominent		OCD made worse	prominent or made worse by atypicals. Sulpiride has been specifically found helpful for tics				
Psychosis	Sertraline Paroxetine if depressive component	If sleep is difficult and agitation is prominent	Venlafaxine for depressive psychosis	Diazepam for insomnia and agitation	1st line: Olanzapine Risperidone Quetiapine Clozapine for treatment resistant (3rd or 4th line)	2nd line: Sulpiride Haloperidol	If major affective component is recurrent	If major affective component which is recurrent	No	No
Bipolar disorder	Since many young bipolar are rapid cyclers caution is needed	Since young bipolars are more often rapid cyclers caution is needed	Since young bipolars are more often rapid cyclers caution is needed	Diazepam for Insomnia and agitation	1st line in psychosis whether manic or depressed	Short term use in acute sedation or to avoid using benzodiazepines for sedation agitation, and akathisia	Ist line for prophylaxis and treatment in all but rapid cyclers	1st line in rapid cyclers Sodium Valproate Carbamazepine	No	No
Aggression	Sertraline Fluoxetine Nefazadone Paroxetine **Start low Go slowly**	Amitriptyline	Only if aggression principal manifestation of depression	Diazepam for acute IV sedation Clonazepam is used in acute psychotic excitement	Risperidone Olanzapine if extreme	IV haloperidol for acute sedation	For severe aggression adjuvant to other treatments and treatment in its own right	Carbamazepine in head injured and intellectually impaired	Dexamphetamine Methylphenidate	Clonidine Guanfacine

(Continued)

Table 25.1 (Continued)

Indications by conditions	SSRIs and 5HT$_{2A}$ antagonists	Tricyclics	SNRIS	Benzodiazepines	Atypical antipsychotics	Typical antipsychotics	Lithium	Anticonvulsants	Stimulants	Alpha-2 agonists
Autistic spectrum disorder (used to target obsessions, aggression, overactivity and self-injury — not core autism)	Sertraline Fluoxetine Paroxetine for obsessions, self-injury and aggression	Amitriptyline for anxiety, aggression and insomnia	Venlaflaxine for depression	For short term insomnia and anxiety. Beware of cortical disinhibition	Risperidone Olanzapine if extreme	Haloperidol for IV sedation when aggression is acute and extreme	Lithium for self-injurious behaviour and extreme aggression	Carbamazepine for stereotypy	For comorbid ADHD — especially in Asperger's syndrome	For insomnia, ADHD and tics especially in Asperger's syndrome
ADHD	If comorbid depression	2nd line: Amitriptyline	3rd or 4th line: Venlafaxine	No	Risperidone in very extreme cases	No	No	No	1st line: Methylphenidate Dexamphetamine	Clonidine said to be better with the impulsive aggressive children and those with tics

Footnote: there is variation between countries with regard to licensing of specific medications — in the UK droperidol and thioridazine have recently been withdrawn.

the profile for adverse reactions for psychotropic medications improves the readiness to use them at an earlier stage in the treatment process is likely to grow. The failure to use them for children whose safety and relief from suffering are likely to benefit seems inhumane. Nevertheless, any treatment must be considered in the light of appropriate indications and weighed against possible adverse effects.

Complications and concerns

There are many anxieties, both public and professional, about the use of medications in children and adolescents. Some in the community are concerned about the whole notion of children having psychiatric disorder, let alone medication to treat it. Others are worried that medications are more toxic in children. Still others believe that medications are unnatural. Psychiatric disorder in childhood is commonly believed, even in professional circles, to be less severe and less distressing than in adulthood and therefore the exposure to the risk of side effects unjustified. The belief that strength of character is all that is needed to deal with all personal problems still persists, along with the view that reliance on medication undermines the development of strength of character. The view that taking psychotropic medication predisposes children to taking illicit drugs is increasingly encountered in clinical practice.

Some of the concerns in the medical community are due to a different and quite complex array of issues. These include the induction of adverse reactions such as tardive dyskinesia, dystonia, and akathisia. More subtle concerns include the possible long term distortion of developing neurotransmitter systems and the medicalisation of family distress by treating the child and failing to address the family difficulties. The inappropriate control of unwanted behaviour by parents, using medication, remains a concern to most practitioners. The fear of overdose, especially in depressed adolescents, and the danger of psychotropic addiction more commonly emerge as issues in the management of adolescents. All of these fears arise against a backdrop of beliefs that environmental strategies and non-medical therapies are, or should be, sufficient for all child psychiatric disorders and that these medications do not work.

Perhaps there are more practical issues that should be raised more often; namely that expertise with these medications is difficult to gain unless seeing larger numbers than most practitioners see and that parents may provide an uncomfortable level of coercion to prescribe once it becomes clear to them that the possibility of obtaining psychotropic medication is an option.

Tardive dyskinesia, tardive dystonia, and tardive akathisia

Tardive dyskinesia is a potential problem in young people and in adults. Children with psychosis are more likely to have more years of exposure to psychotropics. Despite this, tardive dyskinesia is extremely uncommon in children, overwhelmingly emerges with treatment withdrawal, and resolves over time. It is even less likely to occur with the recent change of prescribing to the novel antipsychotics. There have been particular concerns for the older adolescent male. However, more recent reviews suggest a less pessimistic picture. Overall, the young are less likely to suffer from these disorders. Less is known about tardive dystonia and tardive akathisia. They are currently thought to be extremely rare.

Neurotransmitter system distortion

There is no evidence of distortion of neurotransmitter systems at this stage, though clearly we need to keep an open mind and to audit our usage of medication. There is little recognition that young people are engaging in widespread, reckless self-manipulation of their own neurotransmitter systems with illicit drugs when faced with distress, often in the form of anxiety or depression, which is prolonged and sometimes inescapable. There is also a growing concern among neuroscientists and evidence that depression and psychosis are damaging to neurotransmitter systems and to neuronal populations if left untreated.

Contributing to the medicalisation of family distress

The medicalisation of family distress via the prescribing of medication to an individual member may occur at any age. In child psychiatry, we usually employ a family based approach simultaneously with the use of any medication. Identifying the problems of each member of the family and of the family system as a whole can be very freeing for a child who has taken the whole responsibility for the family's difficulties. There is, therefore, more danger of this occurring in adult psychiatric practice in which patients are viewed predominantly in an individual treatment frame.

The inappropriate control of unwanted behaviour

Medication may be used as agents of social or interpersonal control, especially by parents. While this is not limited to childhood, children and the elderly are more vulnerable. Clinicians dealing with children need to be on the alert for this sort of abuse, the extreme of which is Munchausen syndrome by proxy (MSBP), now often called fabricated or induced illness (see chapter 18).

Overdose

This is a danger of overdose in all age groups, but especially:

- Older teenagers and younger adults
- The terminally ill with dramatically reduced quality of life and family conflict
- The actively hopeless with no anticipation of support or relief
- Those suffering unrelieved agitation
- Those disinhibited by substance abuse.

The risk of overdose can be reduced by:

- Eliminating the use of tricyclics in the depressed
- Using relatively safe alternatives such as the SSRIs
- Monitoring closely with short scripts and having frequent review so that distress can be endured with the prospect of relief
- In-patient care when their condition warrants.

The danger of addiction

Withdrawal and addiction are much less common in childhood than adulthood. They begin to emerge as difficulties in middle to late adolescence. Although there is always a theoretical risk of psychological dependency, in practice clinicians do not find this a prominent difficulty.

Syndromes of adverse reaction

Of more concern to all is the possibility that we may do harm with psychotropic medications. As with all medications, adverse reactions are real and many. Thankfully they are generally less frequent and less severe than previously. One way of learning the side effects of medication is to memorise long lists of adverse reactions. A more helpful way is to think of clusters of symptoms commonly encountered. We have called these the syndromes of adverse reaction (Table 25.2). They include:

- The sedation syndrome
- The cerebellar syndrome
- The anticholinergic syndrome
- The extrapyramidal syndromes (EPS)
- The neuroleptic malignant syndrome (NMS)
- The serotonergic syndrome
- The lithium toxicity syndrome
- Haemopoeitc depletion syndromes
- The weight escalation syndrome
- Syndrome of inappropriate antidiuretic hormone secretion (SIADH)
- Neuroadaptation syndromes
- Drug interactions.

These groupings can occur across different drug groups. Some of these side effects can occasionally be beneficial or targetted therapeutically, such as drooling of saliva being helped by the dry mouth caused by the anticholinergic effects of say the tricyclics.

The sedation syndrome

This frequently occurs with the cerebellar syndrome. It is characterised by:

- Tiredness
- Fatigue
- At the beginning of sedation there may be paradoxical disinhibition as the cortex is sedated before the limbic and motor systems
- Difficulty staying awake
- Intermittent falling asleep
- Inability to perform usual tasks
- Yawning
- Unduly deep sleep, even sleep apnoea
- Respiratory depression.

Note that yawning, sleep apnoea and respiratory depression suggest suppression of brainstem activity.

The main medications that give rise to the sedation syndromes are:

- The benzodiazepines, for example diazepam especially when used undiluted and given as a bolus
- The anticonvulsants, for example phenytoin
- The tricyclic antidepressants, for example amitriptyline
- The sedative antipsychotics, for example chlorpromazine and thioridazine.

The cerebellar syndrome

This presents like someone who is drunk because alcohol specifically affects the cerebellum:

- A wide based gait
- An unsteady gait
- Slurred speech
- Clumsiness and past pointing
- Gross, ill-defined, sudden movements
- Decreased muscle tone—a slouching slumped posture
- Disinhibited behaviour (there is debate whether disinhibition can arise from cerebellar disruption alone).

Table 25.2 Syndromes of adverse reaction by medication grouping

Syndromes	SSRIs	TCAs	SNRIS	Benzodiazepine	Atypical or novel antipsychotic	Typical antipsychotic	Lithium salts (CO_2 or citrate)	Anticonvulsants	Stimulants	Adrenergic agonists
Sedation syndrome	Uncommon	Very common especially in first week	Uncommon	Very common	Common on high doses	Common	Usually only with toxic levels	Common	Uncommon	Common
Cerebellar syndrome	Rare	In toxic doses only	Rare	Very common	Common on high doses	Common	Usually only with toxic levels	Very common	No	Uncommon
Anticholinergic	No (except nefazadone)	Common initially and on high doses	No	No	Clozapine	Common except for haloperidol and droperidol which are cholinergic	No	No	No	No
Extrapyramidal syndrome	Uncommon	Uncommon	Uncommon	No	Less common but present on high doses, especially parkinsonism and akathisia	Very common	Uncommon	No	No	No
Neuroleptic malignant syndrome	Rare	Rare	No	No	Rare	Uncommon	No	No	No	No
Serotonergic syndrome	Rare	Rare	Rare	No	No	No	No	No	No	No
Lithium toxicity syndrome	No	No	No	No	No	No	Yes — usually in toxic levels	No	No	No
Haemopoietic depletion syndrome	No	Uncommon	No	No	Clozapine	Uncommon	No — actually increased leukocytes	Uncommon	No	No

(Continued)

Table 25.2 (Continued)

Syndromes	SSRIs	TCAs	SNRIS	Benzodiazepine	Atypical or novel antipsychotic	Typical antipsychotics	Lithium salts (CO_2 or citrate)	Anticonvulsants	Stimulants	Adrenergic agonists
Weight escalation syndrome	No	Uncommon	No	No	Very common	Common	Less common	Common	No	No
Syndrome of inappropriate ADH (induced hyponatremia and fluid retention)	Uncommon	Uncommon	Uncommon	No	No	Phenothiazines have uncommonly caused this syndrome	No. Lithium may cause the opposite problem of diabetes insipidus with polyurea	Carbamazepine uncommon	No	No
Neuroadaptation syndrome	Uncommon	Uncommon	Uncommon	Common	Uncommon	Uncommon	Uncommon	Uncommon	Common	Common

The drugs that most commonly give rise to the cerebellar syndrome include:

- The benzodiazepines
- The anticonvulsants
- Lithium.

The anticholinergic syndrome

This may vary from the mild dryness of mouth and blurring of vision which is associated with the commencement of tricyclics, to the raging hypervigilant psychosis of anticholinergic delirium. The syndrome consists of any, or all, of the following:

- Dry mouth
- Blurred vision
- Tachycardia
- Hypotension
- Constipation
- Urinary retention
- A fine accentuated physiological tremor (10 Hz)
- Prolonged cardiac conductive time (QT interval) > 0·42 milliseconds
- Decreased seizure threshold and seizures
- Delirium with psychosis (an anticholinergic psychosis is characterised by being wide eyed and vigilant, with visual and tactile hallucinations and motor overactivity which is responsive to physostigmine).

The medications that can give rise to this include:

- Tricyclics, especially amitriptyline
- Antihistamines
- Antipsychotics, especially thioradizine.

The extrapyramidal syndromes

The pyramidal fibre tracts in the brain control voluntary muscular movements. Alongside these tracts are another set of tracts called extra (meaning outside of) pyramidal tracts.

They control muscle tone and they affect the involuntary movements of the muscles which support voluntary movement.

Acute increase in muscle tone—dystonia The first muscles to be affected are small muscles of the eyes (the "look ups"), the tongue, the jaw, and the hands. If the muscles of the neck are involved on one side only it is called torticollis. If the muscles at the back of the neck are contracting tightly it is referred to as retrocollis. Opisthotonus refers to the arching of the back and neck and may be confused with hysteria. In children generalised dystonia is more common than in adults and can be mistaken for a seizure. It is extremely frightening for children and their parents. If it involves the laryngeal and pharyngeal muscles it may also be very dangerous. Fortunately, this is rare.

The most common time for acute dystonia to occur is when the medication, usually an antipsychotic or antiemetic, is rising and within the first 5 days, usually the second or third day. It is also more likely to occur in the afternoon or evening. It is usually caused by conventional antipsychotics, high dose atypical antipsychotics, occasionally caused by serotonin selective re-uptake inhibitors (SSRIs) or serotonin and noradrenaline reuptake inhibitors (SNARIs) inhibiting dopamine in the basal ganglia by the elevating serotonin. Serotonin inhibits dopamine in the nigrostriatal pathways.

One of the most common causes is antiemetics such as metoclopramide. Anticholinergic drugs (biperiden, benzatropine mesylate, and procyclidine) and benzodiazepines prevent and treat dystonias. This is one reason why in acute intravenous sedation we use droperidol combined with diazepam.

Psychological and motor restlessness—akathisia Akathisia comes from the Greek meaning "inability to sit down". The tendency to stand up immediately after sitting, and to have an expression of desperation in search of relief upon the face, to communicate by bodily movement a relentlessly compelling sense of discomfort, are all characteristic of akathisia. It is intensely distressing and is difficult to distinguish from the primary agitation of psychosis. In its extreme form the patient has a tormented sense of looking to go somewhere but knowing not where. It most often begins in the early days of commencing a medication but may occur at any time. Rarely it commences after 3 months and is known as tardive akathisia. Akathisia is associated with increased doses and relieved by dose reduction, propanolol (when akathisia is not associated with parkinsonism), anticholinergic agents, and diazepam (when akathisia is associated with parkinsonism). By contrast, psychotic agitation is relieved by increasing doses and recommences as drug levels fall. Any change of medication should be followed by at least 3 days, and where possible longer, to assess the impact of the change and to allow for withdrawal-emergent akathisia.

Drug induced Parkinsonism This usually commences after 5–10 days but unusually may be as late as 3 months of treatment and is characterised by:

- A coarse 3 cycle per second tremor
- Fatigue and anergia
- An expressionless mask-like face
- Flexed posture
- Poverty and slowness of movement (bradykinesia)
- Failure to swing the arms
- Tendency to shuffle the feet in shorter steps (marche à petit pas)
- Hurrying gait (festination)
- A rigidity of arms and legs—especially sometimes referred to as "cogwheel rigidity" or "lead pipe rigidity"
- Increased salivation—sialorrhoea
- Difficulty initiating movement
- Loss of pitch, power and prosidy of speech
- Relief by anticholinergics
- More common in those with lean body mass for example anorexic girls.
- Much less common with the atypical neuroleptics but still occurs, especially at higher doses and especially with risperidone.

A coarse perioral tremor—the rabbit syndrome The combination of the jaw muscles and lip muscles moving together repetitively in tremor produces an appearance resembling the rapid chewing of rabbits. It is actually part of the parkinsonion spectrum of movement disorder and tends to appear after weeks to months and is rare in children and adolescents.

The late onset movement disorder—tardive dyskinesia (TD)
Sometimes young people develop symptoms and signs after months or years. "Tardive" means delayed or late. The features of this condition include:

- Repetitive movements of the mouth and tongue (orobuccal and orolingal dyskinesia).
- May also involve the limbs and trunk.
- Sometimes this gives a twisting, very slow writhing quality which may be more accurately described as tardive dystonia.
- Is usually helped in the short term by increasing the dose but in the longer term by cessation.
- Tetrabenazine has been advocated but TD is generally poorly responsive to treatment. Many would now use a novel antipsychotic such as clozapine or olanzapine which will suppress psychotic symptoms and TD and allow time to recover.
- Made worse by anticholinergics.
- Is very infrequent in children and less common in adolescents, emerges with treatment withdrawal and dissipates with cessation of medication. There have been concerns that older adolescent males were especially at risk although this is now less certain.

Tardive dystonia This is one of the common variants of tardive dyskinesia. Torticollis, retrocollis, blephorospasm and jaw dystonia (Meige's syndrome) are the most common presentations. It is sometimes treated by local botulinum injection into the dystonic muscle groups. Again it is extremely rare in children and disappears with cessation of medication. Despite this rarity, because of the difficulties of older adolescents atypical antipsychotics are the drugs of first line for psychosis in children and adolescents.

The neuroleptic malignant syndrome (NMS)

This is a rare disorder in children and young people characterised by:

- A recent history of antipsychotic exposure
- Confusion moving to unconsciousness
- High or unstable temperatures without infection
- Unduly fluctuating pulse, blood pressure and autonomic nervous system function
- Diaphoresis—profound sweating
- Muscle rigidity
- Elevated creatine phosphokinase (CPK)
- A significant mortality, although precise mortality figures in younger age groups are not known.

The serotonergic syndrome

In its extreme form this is extremely rare in childhood but it may increase in incidence with increased use of serotonergic agents, especially multiple agents. It is essentially the same as the neuroleptic malignant syndrome. However, there is a serotonergic spectrum from mild to severe, with the following characteristics:

- Restlessness and agitation
- Diaphoresis
- Tachycardia
- Headaches
- Shivering or shaking
- Tremor
- Diarrhoea, abdominal cramps, and nausea
- Hyperreflexia
- Hypomania
- Ataxia and incoordination
- Confusion
- Seizures.

These latter difficulties require urgent attention. The advice to patients and parents is if the child becomes sweaty, confused, overactive or looks sick for no apparent reason, present to hospital immediately. Less common side effects that may confuse include swollen lymph nodes, sore joints, dystonias (with neck pain), and nocturnal myoclonic seizures.

Decreased urination, nausea, malaise, lethargy, muscle cramps, seizures and confusion may suggest the syndrome of inappropriate antidiuretic hormone (SIADH) secretion. Death is a serious possibility in these circumstances.

The lithium toxicity syndrome

Lithium is one of the most abundant metals on the Earth's surface and is closely related to sodium in reactivity. The body has difficulty distinguishing lithium from sodium, especially within the kidneys. On hot days we sweat sodium from our skin and concentrate lithium in the body. However, if we have a large meal of chips with a lot of salt, our kidneys will try to get rid of lithium just as much as sodium. The clinical features of acute lithium toxicity are:

- Nausea
- Vomiting
- Diarrhoea
- Tremor
- Hypertonicity, i.e. increased muscle tone
- Delirium
- Seizures
- Cardiac instability.

All this may occur at levels within the therapeutic range but this is unusual. When it does occur, it is frequently associated with neurological disease, multiple medications, or big peak–trough variations. Lithium has a very narrow therapeutic range and in children this is sometimes lower than adults. For acute administration in children doses between 0·8 and 1·00 millimoles per litre are desirable while chronic administration will be between 0·5 and 8·0 millimoles per litre. It is uncommon to get acute toxicity below 0·8 millimoles per litre. Diarrhoea can be reduced by using lithium citrate syrup in children.

Chronic lithium toxicity includes diabetes insipidus (again often dose related) and hypothyroidism and increased neutrophil count.

The haemopoietic depletion syndrome

While lithium may increase white cells and 5-OH tryptophan may increase eosinophils and give a chronic fatigue picture (eosinophilic myalgic syndrome), the most worrying haematopoietic effects of psychotropics are suppression of marrow function and depletion of white cell production in particular. The most serious form of this is agranulocytosis. While it can be caused by the old or typical antipsychotics and the tricyclic antidepressants, the most worrying association is with clozapine usage. This association is worrying because clozapine has been a life saving drug psychiatrically to many and works where so many others have failed. It is more likely to cause blood problems in the elderly and the unwell. Anyone on clozapine requires regular haemopoetic monitoring. The first sign of agranulocytosis might be a sore throat that will not get better.

The syndrome of inappropriate antidiuretic hormone secretion (SIADH)

Although this syndrome is usually described in relation to head trauma, neurosurgery, or central nervous system pathology like abscess, encephalitis, brain tumours, it may also be drug induced. Carbamazepine, the phenothiazines and (more recently described) the SSRIs and tricyclics may lead to this picture. Clinical features include:

- Nausea
- Headache
- Malaise
- Confusion
- Coma
- Seizures
- Low urine output
- Weight gain.

Most of these features are due to fluid overload and cerebral oedema. Serum sodium is low, urine is extra concentrated and low volume. It is usually managed by fluid restriction, electrolyte replacement and very accurate fluid replacement. It requires expert management.

Neuroadaptation syndrome

This is the phenomenon of loss of treatment response sometimes after weeks (acute neuroadaptation) but generally after months of a clear and definite response to medication (chronic or tardive adaptation). The clinician notices that higher and higher doses are required to get the same response but there is no evidence of withdrawal phenomena, i.e. this is not an addiction phenomenon. The best strategy is a period off the particular medication or the use of a drug rotation regimen. It can be deeply distressing to the patient and the family after relief has been gained only to lose it again. Some people refer to this as the "Awakening Response" after the book by Oliver Sacks, or perhaps it should be called the "antiawakening response".

Drug interactions and the cytochrome P450 system in children

The range of medications available to clinicians is so extensive that no clinician can be very familiar with more than a dozen or so medications. However, each clinician needs to know the way these medications interact with the broad range of medications. Key to understanding drug interactions is the understanding of the body's mechanisms for dealing with substances produced both within and outside the body.

The most studied detoxification system in the body is the family of enzymes known as cytochrome P450 (CYP450). Cytochrome P450 is a family of enzymes that deal with toxic substances produced within the body (endogenous) and produced outside of the body (exogenous). The family of enzymes are so big they are referred to as an enzyme superfamily. These enzymes, like all enzymes, are proteins. But they are special because they contain iron in the same way that haemoglobin does. They can utilise oxygen in order to metabolise toxic substances to enable elimination from the body.

Cytochrome P450   There are really only four of relevance for most clinicians—1A2, 2D6, 2C19, 3A4. The liver is the

Table 25.3 Prescribing information on psychotropics in childhood. The doses recommended here are suggestions only and should always be read in conjunction with product information and with due recognition of individual variation. The advice of an experienced colleague should always be sought if using a new medication for the first time

Medication	Indication	Contraindication	Initial dose	Maintenance dose	Maximum dose	Advice, considerations, and side effects
Acamprosate	Maintenance therapy for alcoholism	Renal calculi, pregancy and lactation, renal and hepatic insufficiency	10 mg/kg/day in three divided doses with meals	20 mg/kg/day in three divided doses with meals	25 mg/kg/day	Treatment should last at least 1 year and not be ceased during drinking bouts. Only during severe withdrawal should it be ceased. Tetracyclines may be inactivated by the calcium in the acamprosate. Diarrhoea, nausea, vomiting, abdominal pain, pruritis, maculopapular rashes and occasionally bullous reactions.
Alprazolam	Anxiety, panic, night terrors	History of substance abuse, allergy, psychosis, narrow angle glaucoma	6·25 micrograms/kg/day	25 micrograms/kg/day	For panic 50 micrograms/kg/day	Increases the levels of haloperidol, fluphenazine, astemizole, cisapride, and phenytoin.

(Continued)

Table 25.3 (*Continued*)

Medication	Indication	Contraindication	Initial dose	Maintenance dose	Maximum dose	Advice, considerations, and side effects
						If used concurrently with fluvoxamine, nefazadone, cimetidine, grapefruit juice, fluoxetine or erythromycin, levels will rise. Carbamazepine may lower levels. Addiction in older adolescence
Amitriptyline	ADHD (2nd or 3rd line) anxiety	Hypersensitivity, narrow angle glaucoma, hypomania, mania, caution with seizure disorders, hyperthyroidism, cardiac and liver disease counteracts clonidine.	0·5 mg/kg/day	1·0–1·5 mg/ kg/day at night	1·5 mg/kg/day	Not effective in children and adolescents for depression. May lower seizure threshold. If needed in child with potential for seizures, increase anticonvulsant cover. Interacts with MAOIs, sympathomimetics and cimetidine. Half life up to 24 hours. Anticholinergic syndrome.

(*Continued*)

Table 25.3 (*Continued*)

Medication	Indication	Contraindication	Initial dose	Maintenance dose	Maximum dose	Advice, considerations, and side effects
		Do not use with SSRIs, since SSRIs inhibit the metabolism of tricyclics				
Atenolol	Social phobias withdrawal syndromes, states of high autonomic arousal	Hypersensitivity, hypotensive	1–2 mg/kg/day	2 mg/kg/day	5 mg/kg/day two doses daily	May cause delirium
Benztropine	Extrapyramidal syndromes (short term or 2nd line long term),	Hypersensitivity, narrow angle glaucoma, duodenal obstruction,	0·02 mg/kg/dose If acute EPSE 0·03 mg/kg/	0·02 mg/kg/dose morning and evening If acute	0·03 mg/kg/dose morning and evening If acute	May exacerbate confusion in organic brain syndromes and the intellectually impaired. May still be

(Continued)

Table 25.3 (*Continued*)

Medication	Indication	Contraindication	Initial dose	Maintenance dose	Maximum dose	Advice, considerations, and side effects
	dystonia, akathisia, parkinsonism	severe confusion, (use diazepam in sedation)	dose IV or IM	EPSE 0·03 mg/kg/ dose IV or IM	EPSE 0·03 mg/kg/ dose IV or IM up to 3 doses in 24 hours	necessary to give in an organic brain syndrome. The need is partially obviated by use of benzodiazepines for sedation. Note: IV infusions should be given over 1–2 minutes. Half life greater than 24 hours. Sedation is a common side effect along with headaches, nausea, listlessness, and numbness
Biperiden	Extrapyramidal syndromes (short term or 1st line long term), dystonia, akathisia, parkinsonism	Hypersensitivity, narrow angle glaucoma, duodenal obstruction, severe confusion (use diazepam in sedation)	0·02 mg/kg/ dose If acute EPSE 0·3 mg/kg/ dose IV or IM	0·02–0·4 mg/ kg/day If acute EPSE 0·03 mg/kg/ dose IV or IM	0·06 mg/kg/day If acute EPSE 0·3 mg/kg/dose IV or IM up to three times in 24 hours	May exacerbate confusion in organic brain syndromes and the intellectually impaired. May still be necessary to give in an organic brain syndrome. The need is partially obviated by use of

(*Continued*)

Table 25.3 (*Continued*)

Medication	Indication	Contraindication	Initial dose	Maintenance dose	Maximum dose	Advice, considerations, and side effects
						benzodiazepines for sedation. Give with food to avoid GIT upset. Mild stimulant usually and only occasionally sedates. Note: IV infusions should be given over 1–2 minutes. Half life up to 24 hours. Anticholinergic which is highly selective for the muscarinic receptors. Anticholinergic syndrome
Bromo criptine	Neuroleptic malignant syndrome, cocaine withdrawal, akinetic mutism, sustained hypoactive delirium	Organic delusional syndrome, mania, organic anxiety syndrome	2·5 mg three times a day	10 mg three times a day	1·0 mg/kg/day	Headache, restlessness, abnormal involuntary movements, gastrointestinal upset and hypotension may occur

(*Continued*)

Table 25.3 (Continued)

Medication	Indication	Contraindication	Initial dose	Maintenance dose	Maximum dose	Advice, considerations, and side effects
Buspirone	Anxiety, mixed anxiety-depression, aggression, self-injury	Hypersensitivity, psychosis	2·5 mg twice daily	0·5 mg/kg/day	< 12 years 20 mg; 12–13 years 30 mg; > 13 years 60 mg	Do not use with monoamine oxidase inhibitors. Abdominal pain can occur especially if dose is too high or increments are too frequent or large
Carbamazepine	Bipolar disorder, complex partial and tonic clonic seizures, trigeminal neuralgia, chronic or idiopathic dystonias	Stevens–Johnson syndrome	5 mg/kg/day three or four times a day regimen	10–30 mg/kg/day three or four times a day	< 12 years 1000 mg; > 12 years 1200 mg	Interacts with SSRIs. Autoinduces own metabolism. Blood levels do not always correlate with symptom improvement. *Therapeutic range 26–40 micromoles/litre.* Agranulocytosis 3 × normal population
Chloral hydrate	Short term sedation in under twelves	Renal or hepatic impairment	20 mg/kg/dose	Short term use only 10 mg/kg/day	75 mg/kg/dose	Prolonged use may cause renal or hepatic damage
Citalopram	Depression, anxiety, panic disorder	Hypomania, mania	0·3 mg/kg/day morning or evening	0·5 mg/kg/day in a single dose	0·6 mg/kg/day in a single dose	The most selective of the SSRIs. Treatment emergent

(Continued)

Table 25.3 (Continued)

Medication	Indication	Contraindication	Initial dose	Maintenance dose	Maximum dose	Advice, considerations, and side effects
						hypomania is more common problem in adolescence than is generally recognised. Never use with MAOIs and tricyclics. Half life up to 33 hours. Nausea is a common side effect
Clomipramine	Obsessive compulsive disorder, Tourette's (3rd line in combination), phobic states, cataplexy (in narcolepsy), ADHD	Mania, high suicidality, cardiac abnormality	1 mg/kg/day	2 mg/kg/day	3 mg/kg/day	The main indication is now obsessive compulsive disorder. Although it has the best evidence base many clinicians would use fluvoxamine for safety reasons first. Never use with MAOIs and tricyclics. Half life up to 28 hours. Treatment — emergent hypomania is more common problem in adolescence than is generally recognised

(Continued)

Table 25.3 (*Continued*)

Medication	Indication	Contraindication	Initial dose	Maintenance dose	Maximum dose	Advice, considerations, and side effects
Clonazepam	Acute sedation, bipolar disorder, panic disorder, mixed seizure disorder	Hypersensitivity reaction, narrow angle glaucoma, myasthenia gravis	0·1 mg/dose	0·01–0·02 mg/kg/day in two or three divided doses	2 mg/dose 0·2 mg/kg/day	Long acting benzodiazepine. Remember respiratory depression, the possibility of accumulation and behavioural disinhibition. In the sedated child increased bronchial secretions may cause respiratory pooling
Clonidine	ADHD (2nd line), Tourette's, aggression, akathisia, anxiety, PTSD (1st line for mild symptoms where sedation is also required or high arousal is present)	Hypersensitivity, hypotension, depression, cardiovascular disease	2 micrograms/kg/dose (single evening dose)	5 micrograms/kg/day A twice a day regimen is often used with a loading towards the night	5 micrograms/kg/day	It stimulates the brake on norepinephrine (noradrenaline). Depression occurs in about 5% of cases. Sedation is main side effect and may last up to 4 weeks but usually less than 2 weeks. Precocious puberty is uncommon but reported. *Most serious side effect is hypertensive rebound*

(*Continued*)

Table 25.3 (*Continued*)

Medication	Indication	Contraindication	Initial dose	Maintenance dose	Maximum dose	Advice, considerations, and side effects
						encephalopathy upon cessation. *If cessation necessary taper over 6 days*
Clozapine	Treatment resistant psychosis, psychosis with tardive dyskinesia	Previous blood dyscrasia, allergy, cardiac disease	125 mg evening dose; use 125 mg increments every 3 days	3–5 mg/kg/day in two divided doses	8 mg/kg/day in divided doses	Atypical or novel antipsychotic. Agranulocytosis 1–2%. Weekly monitoring of blood white cell count for first 18 weeks. Majority of cases develop in first 3 months of treatment. Seizures — dose dependent. Orthostatic hypotension, tachycardia and ECG and cardiac changes have been reported. Induced by smoking and inhibited by fluvoxamine. Smokers may require higher doses of clozapine.

(Continued)

Table 25.3 (*Continued*)

Medication	Indication	Contraindication	Initial dose	Maintenance dose	Maximum dose	Advice, considerations, and side effects
						Those on fluvoxamine may get high dose effects including seizures. Citalopram is not affected. Hypersalivation, delirium, incontinence, myocarditis
Desmopressin (DDAVP; 1-desamino-8-D-arginine-vasopressin)	Nocturnal enuresis > 6 years	Von Willibrand's disease	20 micrograms/day intranasally at bed time	20–40 micrograms. Note: if 20 micrograms is adequate try 10 micrograms	40 micrograms/day	Drug interactions with lithium, epinephrine, (adrenaline) heparin, alcohol, and carbamazepine. Dose dependent increases in Factor VIII and induction of platelet aggregation can occur. If they have a bleeding disorder consider consulting haematologist. Hypertension, ENT and GIT complaints

(Continued)

Table 25.3 (*Continued*)

Medication	Indication	Contraindication	Initial dose	Maintenance dose	Maximum dose	Advice, considerations, and side effects
Dextro-amphetamine	ADHD, conduct disorder narcolepsy, frontal disinhibition	Hypersensitivity to sympathomimetic amines, psychosis, drug abuse, hyperthyroidism, Tourette's syndrome	5 mg morning and midday	15–20 mg/day in three divided doses at approx. 8 a.m., 11 a.m. and 4 p.m.	0·5 mg/kg/day for ADHD up to 30 mg; 1 mg/kg/day for narcolepsy up to 60 mg	Stimulant — dopamine agonist — increases release of noradrenaline, dopamine in cerebral cortex, brainstem and reticular activating system. Children with mental age less than 4·5 years do not generally respond to stimulants. Depression. Loss of appetite. Weight loss. Psychosis
Diazepam	Acute sedation (IV), sedation (oral), acute anxiety, anticonvulsant (short term and	Hypersensitivity reaction, narrow angle glaucoma, myasthenia gravis	0·1–0·9 mg/kg/day	For anxiety: under 12 years 10 mg/dose; over 12 years 20 mg/dose	Under 12 years 40 mg/day; over 12 years 60 mg/day	*IV diazepam should not be given in a bolus form but diluted in saline by 20:1 or 25:1, i.e. 10 mg of diazepam in 2 ml in 40–50 ml of saline and given over 5 minutes.*

(*Continued*)

Table 25.3 (*Continued*)

Medication	Indication	Contraindication	Initial dose	Maintenance dose	Maximum dose	Advice, considerations, and side effects
	status epilepticus)					This avoids respiratory depression. Notes 1: antidote to diazepam is flumazenil. Takes approximately 30 minutes to *establish* sedation but will not usually *maintain* sedation beyond 2 hours. Note 2: diazepam is used for anxiety for days to weeks not months to years. Respiratory depression. Bronchial secretion. Idiosyncratic allergy
Droperidol	Acute sedation (IV), acute psychosis	Hypersensitivity, blood dyscrasias, tardive dyskinesia	0·1–0·3 mg/kg/ dose may need to be given every 4–6 hours	0·3 mg/kg dose may need to be given every 4–6 hours	Under 12 years 10 mg/dose over 12 years 20 mg/dose	Typical antipsychotic — butyrophenone. Use in combination with diazepam or benztropine mesylate to avoid extrapyramidal side effects which are more common in children and adolescents.

(Continued)

Table 25.3 (*Continued*)

Medication	Indication	Contraindication	Initial dose	Maintenance dose	Maximum dose	Advice, considerations, and side effects
						Note 1: avoid boluses to reduce hypotension. Dilute 10 mg in 40 ml of saline and give over 5 minutes. Note 2: diazepam is used to establish the sedation while droperidol maintains it for 4–6 hours NB: withdrawn in UK
Flumazenil	Reversal of benzodiazepine toxicity	Hypersensitivity overdosage on tricyclics	0·2 mg IV dose over 30 seconds	2–10 micrograms/kg/ hour	Infusion 3 mg/hour	This drug is a benzodiazepine receptor antagonist
Fluoxetine	Depression, anxiety, obsessive compulsive disorder, bulimia, premenstrual dysphoric disorder, aggression, self-	Hypersensitivity, MAOIs, hypomania, mania, liver Impairment	0·15 mg/kg/day every morning	0·3 mg/kg/day	0·6 mg/kg/day	This SSRI has more evidence for its use in childhood than any other because of its early dominance of the market share. The difficulty is its extraordinarily long half life which, with its active metabolite norfluoxetine, lasts up to 16 days. It

(Continued)

Table 25.3 (Continued)

Medication	Indication	Contraindication	Initial dose	Maintenance dose	Maximum dose	Advice, considerations, and side effects
	injurious behaviour					may take 4–6 weeks to reach steady state levels in the blood. For this reason the recommended washout period if changing from fluoxetine to an MAOI is 4–6 weeks. Agitation, anxiety, nervousness, insomnia, drowsiness, weight loss, diarrhoea, GIT disturbance, skin rash, lowering of seizure threshold are all possible. Flattening of T waves, cardiac conduction difficulties and mild dysrhythmias have been reported. Despite having a greater evidence base those SSRIs with predictable kinetics are easier to manage clinically.

(Continued)

Table 25.3 (Continued)

Medication	Indication	Contraindication	Initial dose	Maintenance dose	Maximum dose	Advice, considerations, and side effects
						Treatment — emergent hypomania is more common problem in adolescence than is generally recognised. Vasculitis has been recorded. *Half life up to 140 hours and active metabolite norfluoxetine up to 16 days*
Fluvoxamine	Depression, anxiety, obsessive compulsive (FDA approval for 8–12 years old) disorder (lst line), aggression, self-injurious behaviour	Hypersensitivity, hypomania, mania, MAOIs, liver impairment	1 mg/kg/day in two divided doses	2 mg/kg/day in two divided doses	3 mg/kg/day in two divided doses	Mildly sedating and nauseating so the dosage may be greater at bed time. Treatment — emergent hypomania is a more common problem in adolescence than is generally recognised. Hyponatraemia. Inhibits P450 enzymes *moderately to strongly.* Half life up to 22 hours

(Continued)

Table 25.3 (Continued)

Medication	Indication	Contraindication	Initial dose	Maintenance dose	Maximum dose	Advice, considerations, and side effects
Haloperidol (also available in depot form —decanoate)	Psychosis (2nd or 3rd line treatment), acute sedation, Tourette's syndrome (2nd line in children although still argued by some to be 1st line), extreme ADHD unresponsive to other measures	Hypersensitivity, blood dyscrasias, bone marrow depression, withdrawal states, previous history of EPSE especially akathisia	0·035 mg in two divided doses	0·07–0·2 mg/ kg/day in two divided doses	0·2 mg/kg/day in two divided doses	Typical antipsychotic — butyrophenone. *Inhibition of conversion of codeine to morphine.* Lithium does not combine well with haloperidol and may lead to encephalopathy. Poor diabetic control due to interaction with insulin and oral hypoglycemics. SSRIs may increase risk of EPSEs
Imipramine	Enuresis, ADHD, *not for depression in children and adolescents*	Hypersensitivity, narrow angle glaucoma, hypomania, mania, caution	0·5 mg/kg/day	1·0–1·5 mg/kg/ day night time dose	100 mg/day	Tricyclic with greater noradrenergic effects. Do not use with SSRIs since SSRIs inhibit the metabolism of tricyclics.

(Continued)

Table 25.3 (Continued)

Medication	Indication	Contraindication	Initial dose	Maintenance dose	Maximum dose	Advice, considerations, and side effects
		with seizure disorders, hyperthyroidism and cardiac disease counteracts clonidine				*Not effective in children and adolescents for depression.* May lower seizure threshold. If needed in child with potential for seizures increase anticonvulsant cover. Half life up to 18 hours. Urinary retention
Lamotrigine	Bipolar disorder where valproate, lithium or carbamazepine is ineffective or unable to be used and depression is prominent. Acute mania, prophylaxis, rapid cycling, adjunctive	Pregnancy and lactation, hepatic impairment	0.3–0.5 mg/kg/ day. Increase slowly every 2 weeks in 25 mg increments. Establish twice daily dosing	10–15 mg/kg/ day	Maximum 700 mg/day or if on valproate 5 mg/kg/day	Blocks release of glutamate and aspartate and inactivates sodium channels leading to reduction of repetitive neuronal firing. Valproate increases half life to up to 60 hours. Carbamazepine, phenytoin, phenobarbital, primidone (inducers) reduce half life to around 15 hours. Lamotrigine decreases carbamazepine sometimes dramatically.

(Continued)

Table 25.3 (*Continued*)

Medication	Indication	Contraindication	Initial dose	Maintenance dose	Maximum dose	Advice, considerations, and side effects
	treatment for partial epilepsy and generalised seizures					Half life around 24 hours. Dizziness, diplopia, sleepiness, headache, ataxia, weakness and fatigue, nausea, rash. Disseminated intravascular coagulation. Do not stop suddenly — to avoid withdrawal seizures discontinue over 2–4 week period. Stevens–Johnson and other severe rashes may occur
Lithium	Bipolar disorder, aggression, conduct disorder, depressive	Renal damage, thyroid disease. Caution in the intellectually impaired and	125 mg twice a day and titrate against serum levels taken each week and	Acute bipolar episode trough serum levels of 0·8–1·0 millimoles per litre	Acute bipolar episode trough, serum levels of 0·8–1·0 millimoles	Baseline renal, thyroid and blood film. Avoid haloperidol and lithium together. Avoid carbemazepine and lithium together.

(Continued)

Table 25.3 (*Continued*)

Medication	Indication	Contraindication	Initial dose	Maintenance dose	Maximum dose	Advice, considerations, and side effects
	treatment adjuvant	organically impaired, children with parents who are chaotic and unreliable, *pregnancy*	monitoring for adverse effects on a second daily basis	maintenance; bipolar 0·6–0·8 millimoles per litre; all other 0·5–0·7 millimoles per litre.	per litre maintenance; bipolar 0·6–0·8 millimoles per litre; all other 0·5–0·7 millimoles per litre	Half life up to 20 hours. Polyurea and polydipsia may develop and are usually relieved by lowering the dose. Tremor is the most noticeable problem. This is improved by lower doses and propanolol where extreme. Acne may be problematic for adolescents. *Trough levels need to be taken approximately 12 hours after last dose*
Lorazepam	Acute sedation (IM). Note: IM is unavailable in Australia	Hypersensitivity to benzodiazepines, narrow angle glaucoma	IV sedation 0·044 mg/kg/ dose given slowly over 3 minutes, titrate against response	Not applicable	2 mg IV over 3 minutes	Benzodiazepine. Note: antidote to benzodiazepine is flumazenil. Orthostatic hypotension

(Continued)

Table 25.3 (Continued)

Medication	Indication	Contraindication	Initial dose	Maintenance dose	Maximum dose	Advice, considerations, and side effects
Methylphenidate	ADHD, conduct disorder, frontal disinhibition, narcolepsy (1st line stimulant)	Hypersensitivity to sympathomimetic-amines, psychosis, drug abuse, hyperthyroidism, Tourette's syndrome	10 mg morning and evening	30–40 mg/day in three divided doses at approx. 8 a.m., 11 a.m. and 4 p.m.	1·0 mg/kg/day for ADHD up to 60 mg; 1 mg/kg/day for narcolepsy up to 60 mg	Dopamine agonist. Children with mental age less than 4·5 years do not generally respond to stimulants. Depression in low or normal doses and psychosis in high doses have been reported. Loss of appetite. Weight loss
Midazolam	Acute sedation, acute treatment of seizures	Hypersensitivity to benzodiazepines, narrow angle glaucoma	IM 0·2 mg/kg/dose; IV 0·1–0·2 mg/kg/dose	Not applicable	Repeat dose if no response in 2 minutes	Benzodiazepine. Oral, IM and IV doses. Medazalam is usually adequate to establish a sedation but not to maintain it unless in an intensive care setting
Mirtazapine	Depression (3rd line)	Hypersensitvity, caution in those with history of bipolar disorder	0·1 mg/kg/day	0·2–0·5 mg/kg/day as a single night time dose	0·5 mg/kg/day	5HT$_{2A}$ antagonist Avoid alcohol. Do not combine with MAOIs. Half life up to 40 hours. Minimal drug interaction.

(Continued)

Table 25.3 (Continued)

Medication	Indication	Contraindication	Initial dose	Maintenance dose	Maximum dose	Advice, considerations, and side effects
						Drowsiness. Weight gain. Seizures. LFTs may be affected. Oedema
Moclobemide	Social phobia, anxiety, depression, panic, ADHD	Hypomania, mania, *concurrent use of "ecstasy" (i.e. MDMA)*	1 mg/kg/day once a day in morning dose	3–4 mg/kg/day in two divided doses morning and afternoon	6 mg/kg/day	Reversible inhibitor of monooxidase A, i.e. RIMA. Low rate of side effects. Dry mouth, dizziness, headaches, restlessness, insomnia, rash, nausea and occasionally sedation. Given 1 hour after meals will reduce headaches. Morning and afternoon dosage will reduce insomnia. *Tricyclics, SSRIs, sympathomimetics, cimetidine, L-DOPA, sumatryptan and narcotics should not be used at the same time.*

(Continued)

Table 25.3 (Continued)

Medication	Indication	Contraindication	Initial dose	Maintenance dose	Maximum dose	Advice, considerations, and side effects
						2 weeks needed for washout of tricyclics and SSRIs. Treatment — emergent hypomania is more common problem in adolescence than is generally recognised. Half life up to 2 hours
Naltrexone	Self-injurious behaviour in autistic spectrum disorder and intellectually impaired alcohol dependence (reduces craving and increases abstinence)	Hypersensitivity, acute withdrawal from opiates, concomitant use of opioids	0·5 mg/kg/day in two or three divided doses	2–3 mg/kg/day in two or three divided doses	3 mg/kg/day in two or three divided doses	Opiate antagonist. Sedation. Evidence is not strong for efficacy in self-injurious behaviour

(Continued)

Table 25.3 (*Continued*)

Medication	Indication	Contraindication	Initial dose	Maintenance dose	Maximum dose	Advice, considerations, and side effects
Nefazadone	Depression, mixed anxiety and depression	Hypersensitvity, caution in those with history of orthostatic hypotension or bipolar disorder	0·5 mg/kg/day in single evening dose	2–4 mg/kg/day in two divided doses	6 mg/kg/day in two divided doses	Serotonin 2A antagonist and mild reuptake inhibitor of noradrenaline and serotonin. *Powerful inhibitor of CYP3A4 enzymes.* Do not use with RIMAs or traditional MAOIs. Alprazalam levels are likely to rise on this drug. Half life of 4 hours. Headache, nausea, somnolence, dry mouth, dizziness, light headedness, insomnia, constipation are all common. Treatment — emergent hypomania is more common problem in adolescence than is generally recognised.

(*Continued*)

Table 25.3 (Continued)

Medication	Indication	Contraindication	Initial dose	Maintenance dose	Maximum dose	Advice, considerations, and side effects
Olanzapine	Psychosis (1st line), schizophrenia, bipolar disorder,	Hypersensitivity	0·1 mg/kg/day in two divided doses	0·1–0·2 mg/ kg/day in two divided doses	0·25 mg/kg/day	Atypical antipsychotic thienobenzodiazepine — antagonist of dopamine and serotonin $5HT_{2A}$. Metabolised by enzymes which are induced by smoking and and carbamazepine and inhibited by fluvoxamine. Smokers may require slightly higher doses of olanzapine. Those on fluvoxamine may get high dose effects. *Weight gain with striae,* sedation, hypotension, anticholinergic effects and changes in liver function tests. Extrapyramidal side effects in higher doses
Paroxetine	Depression, anxiety, obsessive	Hypersensitivity, hypomania, mania,	0·2 mg/kg/day in two divided doses	0·35 mg/kg/day in two divided doses	0·5 mg/kg/day in two divided doses for	Selective serotonin reuptake inhibitor *Withdraw slowly.*

(Continued)

Table 25.3 (*Continued*)

Medication	Indication	Contraindication	Initial dose	Maintenance dose	Maximum dose	Advice, considerations, and side effects
	compulsive disorder (Ist line), panic, social phobia, aggression, self-injurious behaviour	liver impairment, MAOIs			depression 0·6 mg/kg/day	Half life up to 24 hours but may be considerably shorter in adolescents and children and withdrawal reactions occur more frequently. Mildly sedating and nauseating so the dosage may be greater at bed time. Treatment — emergent hypomania is more common problem in adolescence than is generally recognised. Hyponatraemia
Physostigmine	Anticholinergic overdose, anticholinergic psychosis	Hypersensitivity	0·02 mg/kg/ over at least two minutes. May be repeated at 10 minute intervals if necessary.		2 mg dose	Do not use unless there is difficulty gaining control using cholinergic antipsychotics such as droperidol and haloperidol. Atropine should be available to reverse effects.

(Continued)

Table 25.3 (*Continued*)

Medication	Indication	Contraindication	Initial dose	Maintenance dose	Maximum dose	Advice, considerations, and side effects
						Physostigmine has a short half life so repeated doses will be necessary every 1–2 hours for the most intense phase of the psychosis. Stomach aches and cardiac dysrhythmia.
Procyclidine	EPSEs (short term and 1st line long term), acute dystonia, akathisia, Parkinsonism	Hypersensitivity, narrow angle glaucoma, duodenal obstruction, severe confusion (use diazepam in acute sedation)	0·1 mg/kg/day in three divided oral doses. If acute EPSE 0·1–0·15 mg/kg/dose IVI or IMI	0·1–0·2 mg/kg/day in three divided oral doses. If acute EPSE 0·1–0·15 mg/kg/dose IVI or IMI	0·25 mg/kg/day in three divided oral doses. If acute EPSE 0·1–0·15 mg/kg/dose up to four doses in a day IVI or IMI	Anticholinergic — reasonably M2 selective. May exacerbate confusion in organic brain syndromes and the intellectually impaired. May still be necessary to give in an organic brain syndrome. The need is partially obviated by use of benzodiazepines for sedation. Mild stimulant. Dizziness and headaches.

(*Continued*)

Table 25.3 (Continued)

Medication	Indication	Contraindication	Initial dose	Maintenance dose	Maximum dose	Advice, considerations, and side effects
						Note: IV infusions should be given over 1–2 minutes.
Propanolol	Anxiety, akathisia (not associated with Parkinsonism), aggression (with marked autonomic arousal)	Asthma and diabetes are relative contraindications only.	0·5–1·0 mg/kg/day in three or four divided doses	2 mg/kg/day in three or four divided doses	160 mg/day	β blocker — non-selective. Monitor blood pressure and warn of orthostatic hypotension. Exercise tolerance will be affected where exercise is prolonged and demanding
Quetiapine	Psychosis	Hypersensitivity	0·25 mg/kg/day in two divided doses	3 mg/kg/day in two divided doses	5 mg/kg/day in two divided doses	Atypical antipsychotic—a dibenzothiazepine. A weak dopamine blocker and $5HT_{2A}$ antagonist. Low interference with prolactin but low antipsychotic potential as well. Hypotension, dry mouth, constipation, weight gain, LFT changes, TFT changes. Caution nefazadone and fluvoxamine. *Sedation*

(Continued)

Table 25.3 (*Continued*)

Medication	Indication	Contraindication	Initial dose	Maintenance dose	Maximum dose	Advice, considerations, and side effects
Reboxetine	Depression (3rd line), social phobia	Hypersensitivity, hypomania, mania	0·5 mg/kg/day	0·1–0·15 mg/kg/day	0·2 mg/kg/day	Noradrenergic agonist — noradrenaline reuptake inhibitor NARI. Insomnia, sweating, dry mouth, constipation and urinary hesitancy. Do not combine with MAOIs Half life around 13 hours
Risperidone	Psychosis (1st line), severe aggression, Tourette's syndrome (1st line), self-injurious behaviour, ADHD (4th line)	Hypersensitivity to risperidone	0·015 mg/kg/day in two divided doses	0·035 mg/kg/day in two divided doses	0·05 mg/kg/day in two divided doses	Atypical antipsychotic—a benzizoxazole. *Weight gain with striae* which may be worse in adolescents. Akathisia which may be worse in adolescents. Insomnia. Enuresis. Extrapyramidal in higher doses which may be worse in children and adolescents especially when used in

(*Continued*)

Table 25.3 (Continued)

Medication	Indication	Contraindication	Initial dose	Maintenance dose	Maximum dose	Advice, considerations, and side effects
						conjuction with serotonergic medications. Rhinitis and nose bleeds. Sedation. Interacts with SSRIs to cause extrapyramidal reactions. Risperidone clearance increased with carbamazepine
Sertraline	Depression (Ist line), anxiety (Ist line), obsessive compulsive disorder, aggression, self-injurious behaviour	Known hypersensitivity, caution if bipolar history or psychotic depression, do not use if on MAOIs	0·5 mg/kg/day morning dose; 12·5 mg increments every 5–7 days	1·5–2·5 mg/ kg/day morning dose	3 mg/kg/day	SSRI. Akathisia is common in children. GIT disturbances. Rash. Headache. Dystonias, dizzines and tremors. Syndrome of inappropriate antidiuretic hormone. May lower seizure threshold.

(Continued)

Medication	Indication	Contraindication	Initial dose	Maintenance dose	Maximum dose	Advice, considerations, and side effects
						Treatment — emergent hypomania is more common problem in adolescence than is generally recognised. *Inhibits P450 enzymes which can lead to very high levels of tricyclics if used concurrently. Do not use tricyclics and SSRIs in combination.* May lead to extrapyramidal side effects when used concurrently with risperidone. Half life up to 26 hours
Sodium valproate	Bipolar disorder (1st line in young people) and those with mixed affective states or	Hypersensitivity to valproate, *pregnancy,* lactation	10 mg/kg/day in two divided doses	10–20 mg/kg/ day and adjust upwards until *trough* serum levels 500–600 micromoles/ litre	60 mg/kg/day in two divided doses	Takes 2–3 weeks to begin to work and 6–8 weeks to be sure. May increase MAOI and TCA levels. May potentiate the activity of aspirin and warfarin.

(Continued)

Table 25.3 (*Continued*)

Table 25.3 (*Continued*)

Medication	Indication	Contraindication	Initial dose	Maintenance dose	Maximum dose	Advice, considerations, and side effects
	unresponsive to lithium					Short term hair loss — consider zinc supplements. Weight gain. Sedation. Tremor. GIT irritation. Menstrual disturbances. Polycystic ovarian syndrome i.e. hyperandrogenism and chronic anovulation in the absence of underlying pituitary disease. 50% are obese. Young peripubertal girls are most at risk. Clinicians may wish to do baseline ultrasonography. Pancreatitis. Insulin resistance. Hepatotoxicity may occur in the very young,

(Continued)

Table 25.3 (Continued)

Medication	Indication	Contraindication	Initial dose	Maintenance dose	Maximum dose	Advice, considerations, and side effects
						neurodevelopmentally impaired infant on multiple medications. Liver and renal function tests should be done at the outset. Blood dyscrasias, especially thrombocytopenia and neutropenia
Sulpiride	Psychosis (3rd line), where weight gain on atypicals is becoming a major concern.	Hypersensitivity to sulpiride, phaeochromocytoma, Parkinson's disease. **Precautions:** cardiovascular disease; mania or hypomania; hypersensitivity to metoclopramide	6 mg/kg/day in two or three divided doses	10 mg/kg/day in two or three divided doses	20 mg/kg/day	Atypical antipsychotic. Highly selective dopamine 2 blocker. Food interferes with absorption by up to 30%. Sulpiride has a short half life of 6–8 hours. Since sulpiride is a mild antidepressant especially in lower doses it may exacerbate hypomania or mania. Although it is highly D2 specific, extrapyramidal side effects still occur.

(Continued)

Table 25.3 (*Continued*)

Medication	Indication	Contraindication	Initial dose	Maintenance dose	Maximum dose	Advice, considerations, and side effects
						2–6 hours before peak plasma concentration. Weight gain is less than clozapine. if lithium is being used concurrently reduce dosage of lithium
Temazepam	Insomnia	Hypersensitivity to benzodiazepines. Myasthenia gravis. Factors contributing to cortical disinhibition	0·3 mg/kgm/ dose evening	0·3–0·5 mg/kg/dose evening	0·5 mg/kg/dose in any 12 hour period	Small doses are not necessarily safer. Cortical disinhibition of aggression, self-injury and suicidality together with the impulse to flee to a place of safety are all more likely if inadequate doses are used. Along with this occasionally an abreactive response occurs and grief, rejection or histories of abuse may emerge towards the time for sleep

(*Continued*)

Table 25.3 (*Continued*)

Medication	Indication	Contraindication	Initial dose	Maintenance dose	Maximum dose	Advice, considerations, and side effects
Topiramate	Bipolar disorder where valproate, lithium,carbamazepine or lamotrigine are ineffective or unable to be used; acute mania; prophylaxis; rapid cycling; adjunctive treatment for partial epilepsy and secondary generalised seizures; Lennox – Gastaut syndrome; primary tonic clonic seizures	Pregnancy and lactation	1 mg/kg/day 8–12 hourly dosing increase in increments of 1–2 mg/kg/ week	3 mg/kg/day 8–12 hourly dosing	18 mg/kg/day 8–12 hourly dosing	The evidence for use in bipolar disorder is weak. This is an end of the line treatment option for bipolar disorder and requires a combination of expert child psychiatric and neurological expertise. We would recommend this sort of collaboration where possible for commencement of topiramate. Avoid abrupt withdrawal. No clear relationship between trough plasma concentrations and therapeutic response in bipolar disorder has been established. Ensure adequate hydration to prevent nephrolithiasis.

(*Continued*)

Table 25.3 (*Continued*)

Medication	Indication	Contraindication	Initial dose	Maintenance dose	Maximum dose	Advice, considerations, and side effects
	(treatment resistant)					Abdominal pain, nausea, weight loss, confusion, emotional lability, mood disorders, ataxia, dizziness, fatigue, visual disturbances, nystagmus, psychotic symptoms, aggression, and leucopenia
Tranylcypromine	Treatment resistant depression (4th line)	Hypersensitivity, known regular users of "ecstasy", phaeochromocytoma, hyperthyroidism, cautious use in bipolar disorder	0·1 mg/kg/day given in a morning dose	0·15–0·2 mg/kg/day in morning and afternoon doses	0·5 mg/kg/day in morning and afternoon doses	Monoamine oxidase inhibitor. Interactions with opioids, tricyclics, tryptophan, SSRIs, SNARIs, NARIs and venlafaxine. Dizziness, confusion, headache, anxiety, tremor, insomnia, dry mouth, constipation, anorexia, hypotension, hypertensive crisis with tyramine foods and arrhythmias.

(*Continued*)

Table 25.3 (*Continued*)

Medication	Indication	Contraindication	Initial dose	Maintenance dose	Maximum dose	Advice, considerations, and side effects
						Metabolised to amphetamine and may have mild dependence. Half life 2·5 hours
5OH tryptophan	Self-injurious behaviour, treatment resistant obsessive compulsive disorder	Care must be taken with concurrent use of SSRIs to avoid the serotonergic syndrome	100 mg evening	5 mg/kg/day	600 mg/day	Specialist centres only. Should only be commenced if reduced serotonin or 5HIIA in CSF. Reuptake inhibitors will not work in the absence of substrate. They should be retried after 3 months 5OH tryptophan replacement. 5OH trytophan gives tenfold better blood levels than tryptophan. Evidence base in childhood yet to be established. Purest form necessary to avoid eosinophilic myalgia. Pharmaceutical grade best but laboratory grade usually adequate

(*Continued*)

Table 25.3 (*Continued*)

Medication	Indication	Contraindication	Initial dose	Maintenance dose	Maximum dose	Advice, considerations, and side effects
Venlafaxine	Depression, ADHD (4th line)	Hypersensitivity, hypomania, mania, pregnancy	1 mg/kg/day in two or three divided doses or one morning sustained release dose	2–2.5 mg/kg/day in two or three divided doses or one morning sustained release dose	4 mg/kg/day in two or three divided doses or one morning dose if sustained release	Serotonin and noradrenaline selective reuptake inhibitor. Interaction with MAOIs — do not combine. Taken with food. Minor effects on P450 enzymes. Monitor BP twice weekly for period of incremental increases since elevated blood pressure at higher doses. Nausea, insomnia, dry mouth, rash. Very short half life of 5 hours and active metabolite about 11 hours *unless using extended release preparation. Withdrawal effects are common and may even occur with late doses.*

(*Continued*)

Table 25.3 (*Continued*)

Medication	Indication	Contraindication	Initial dose	Maintenance dose	Maximum dose	Advice, considerations, and side effects
						Treatment — emergent hypomania is a more common problem in adolescence than is generally recognised
Zolpiclone	Short term treatment of insomnia in children > 12 years (1st line)	Hypersensitivity to zolpidem	7·5 mg/dose/ day	7·5–15 mg/ dose/day	15 mg/dose/ day	At this point addiction is not thought to be as big a problem as with the benzodiazepines. Do not use under 10 years of age. Use chloral hydrate instead
Zolpidem (an imidazopyridine)	Short term treatment of insomnia in children > 12 years (1st line)	Hypersensitivity to zolpidem	5 mg/dose/day	5–10 mg/dose/ day	10 mg/dose/ day	At this point addiction is not thought to be as big a problem as with the benzodiazepines. Do not use under 10 years of age. Use chloral hydrate instead. Amnesia for period just prior to sleep

(Continued)

Table 25.3 (*Continued*)

Medication	Indication	Contraindication	Initial dose	Maintenance dose	Maximum dose	Advice, considerations, and side effects
Zuclopenthixol	Acute psychosis which is not responsive to other forms of control. (4th line) *Short term usage only*	Hypersensitivity to thioxanthenes or phenothiazines. Organic brain damage especially where this is subcortical, blood dyscrasias, CNS, depression phaeochromo-cytoma *neuroleptic naïve patient*	1 mg/kg/dose (IM) every 3 days or until control is being lost (whichever comes first)	1·5 mg/kg/dose (IM) every 3 days or until control is being lost (whichever comes first). Consideration for conversion to depot or oral medication should take place rather than this being a maintenance regimen	2 mg/kg/dose/ *3 days*	This medication should only be used in young people (postpubertal):- who have had psychotropics before; in whom all else has failed; where there is imminent danger of serious injury to self or others; who have been discussed with an experienced colleague; who are concomitantly prescribed an anticholinergic or a benzodiazepine.

main site of action in humans. Indiana University Medical Centre provides online information on the P450 system (http:/222.Drug-Interactions.com).

Variation in the population There is a variation from slow metabolisers, fast metabolisers to ultrafast metabolisers.

Asians and Afro-Americans are more likely to be slow metabolisers than Caucasians except for 2D6.

Conclusion on drug interaction No one remembers every interaction. It is wise to have information close at hand (Table 25.3) while prescribing, such as that provided by Indiana University. If we can understand what a substrate, an inhibitor and an inducer are, we will understand the process of pharmacokinetics better.

Conclusion

Medication is just one form of treatment in the armamentarium against child psychiatric disorder. It does have a place but neither as limited nor as excessive as some practitioners believe. There is no substitute to discussing medication issues with an experienced person and gaining practical experience in using medications. Understanding the personal significance of prescribing to the child and family, working through adverse effects and adherence issues, together with enhancing the effects of medications with non-biological therapies, are all critical.

Further reading

Green WH. *Child and adolescent clinical psychopharmacology.* Baltimore: Williams and Wilkins, 1995.

Keltner NL, Folks DG. *Psychotropic drugs.* St Louis: Mosby, 1997.

Kutcher SP. *Child and adolescent psychopharmacology.* Philadelphia: WB Saunders, 1997.

Nunn KP, Dey C. *Clinical guidelines for psychotropic usage in childhood.* Department of Psychological Medicine, The Children's Hospital at Westmead, 2002.

Stahl SM. *Essential psychopharmacology.* Cambridge: Cambridge University Press, 2000.

Section IV
The last word

26: The child's view

The book so far has been based on a clinician's perspective. We feel the last word should be that of the child. To this end we present some art work created by children during the course of our contact with them. As with play, artwork can be used by the child to communicate aspirations, inner emotional turmoil and interpersonal conflict where words seem inadequate and where conscious auditing is bypassed. Art is a safe medium to explore inner experiences and their underlying dynamics, and can subsequently facilitate the process of healing. It is particularly useful for children and adolescents as they often lack the verbal sophistication of adults yet find themselves at ease with art as a means of expression.

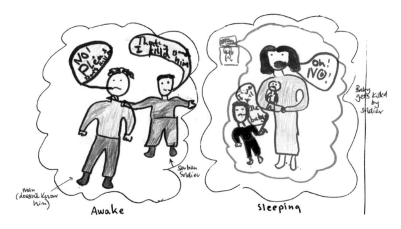

Figure 26.1a

Figure 26.1a: Drawing by ten year old girl with post traumatic stress disorder following atrocities experienced in Kosovo. The pictures represent re-experience of killings; the left picture is of a "flashback" showing a man being killed, while that on the right is of a nightmare depicting a soldier killing a baby.

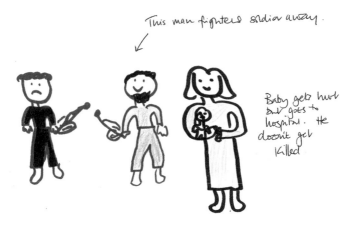

This man fightets sldia away.

Baby gets hurt but goes to hospital. He doesn't get killed

Figure 26.1b

Figure 26.1b: In treatment, the same ten year old girl was asked to change the ending of her nightmare. She described drawing a man who frightens away a murderer so that a baby does not get killed. This "rewriting" of her dream, and regaining of control in her dream world resulted in reduced frequency of flashbacks and nightmares.

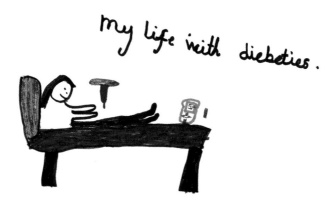

my life with diebeties.

Figure 26.2

Figure 26.2: Drawing by seven year old girl with diabetes who administers her own medication. She drew the picture to show her doctor what her life was like with diabetes.

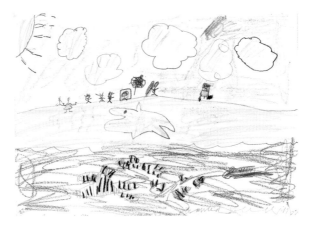

Figure 26.3

Figure 26.3: Drawing by a six year old with school refusal secondary to bullying. The drawing is of several sharks in the sea and one on the beach.

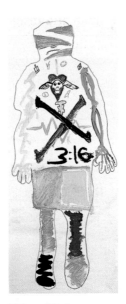

Figure 26.4

Figure 26.4: 15 year old boy with Crohn's disease and colectomy. He stated that the cross overlying the "life line" on his abdomen represents his fight with illness. The bandage covering his head represents his view that he needed protection from the outside world.

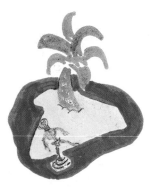

Figure 26.5

Figure 26.5: Adolescent, with inflammatory bowel disease, ambivalent about accepting treatment with resultant weight loss. He explained his skeletal body is on a desert island because he feels isolated, small and insignificant.

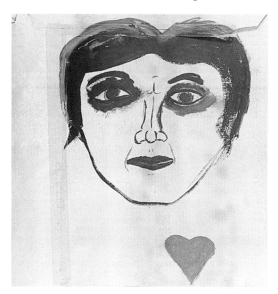

Figure 26.6

Figure 26.6: Self portrait by adolescent boy with depression. He said the predominance of black, particularly around the eyes, represented sadness, boredom and fatigue. He explained that the only reference to his body was a heart because he could not draw a body that suited his face.

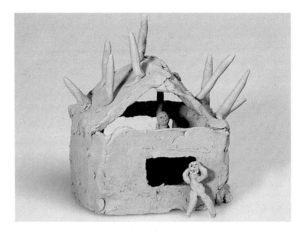

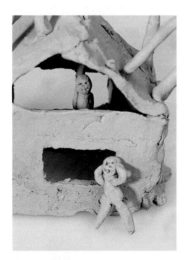

Figure 26.7

Figure 26.7: Clay model by 14 year old boy who displayed long term suicidal ideation. He said that the model was of a hermit hanging inside a home with spikes on the roof, with a shocked observer looking in through the window. He explained that the spikes were there to keep people out, but the hermit became so lonely and insane that he hung himself.

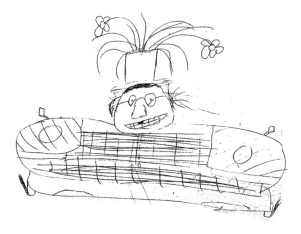

Figure 26.8

Figure 26.8: Self portrait by 14 year old boy with separation anxiety disorder and Asperger syndrome. He said he drew his face attached to his mother's car. He explained that his mother "drives him mad". He drew flowers coming out of his head and potatoes emerging from his ears because his mother likes gardening.

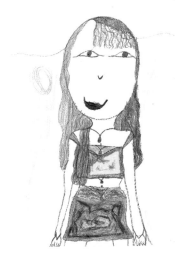

Figure 26.9

Figure 26.9: Self portrait by eight year old with obsessive compulsive disorder. She said she tried very hard to keep the colours within the lines.

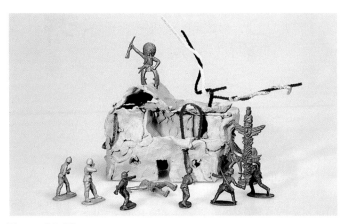

Figure 26.10

Figure 26.10: Clay model of a perceived ideal home by a child with disruptive behaviour. He has depicted his home as a war zone with soldiers fighting outside. He described dreams about converting his home into a two storey building, with him living in the upper part and his parents living in the lower part. This coincided with a strong expressed desire on his part to become more independent of his parents.

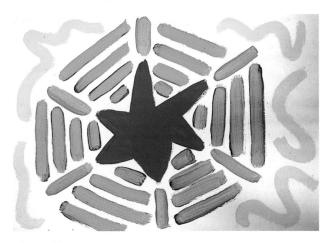

Figure 26.11

Figure 26.11: Adolescent with anorexia nervosa. She desribed the blue star trapped in a maze as representing her anger and the difficulties in accessing and expressing it.

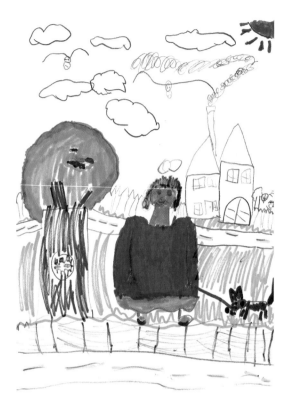

Figure 26.12

Figure 26.12: Self portrait of six year old girl with obesity who represents herself considerably larger than she is in reality. Note the size of her body when compared to the tree and dog.

Acknowledgements

We are extremely grateful to the children and adolescents and their parents for granting permission to reproduce their artwork in this section and on the cover.

Index

Note: Page numbers in **bold** refer to figures and those in *italics* refer to tables or boxed material. Common abbreviations used in sub entries include; ADHD, attention deficit hyperactivity disorder; OCD, obsessive compulsive disorder; PTSD, post-traumatic stress disorder and SSRIs, selective serotonin reuptake inhibitors.